CONTENTS

Introduction 4

The Uncle Ben's
7-Day Rice Diet® 7

Main Dishes 30

Side Dishes 65

Salads 91

Desserts 117

Index 124

INTRODUCTION

Ordering fish instead of steak? Passing up the corn chips? Saying no to desserts? If so, you're part of a growing trend that is changing the way America eats. Today's menus are lighter and leaner, but their emphasis on fresh produce, grains, poultry and fish makes them no less satisfying.

The U.S.D.A. Dietary Guidelines for Americans advise limiting foods which are high in fat, cholesterol and sodium, and eating more foods which are rich in complex carbohydrates such as fruits, vegetables and grains. In fact, the American Dietetic Association recommends that 50 to 60 percent of the calories in the diet each day come from complex carbohydrates.

Rice, one of the world's most popular and versatile grains, is an excellent source of complex carbohydrates.

EATING RIGHT WITH RICE

UNCLE BEN'S® CONVERTED® Brand Rice contains no fat, cholesterol or sodium and just 100 calories per half-cup serving.

Uncle Ben's uses a special processing method before milling which forces vitamins and minerals contained in the outer bran layer toward the center of the rice grain. As a result, after milling, UNCLE BEN'S® Rice contains twice the amount of natural B-complex vitamins as ordinary milled rice. The special processing method also removes the excess surface starch which can make ordinary milled rice sticky. UNCLE BEN'S® Rice remains separate and firm, even when cooked ahead, refrigerated or frozen and reheated.

The Uncle Ben's 7◊Day Rice Diet®

Plus 120 Easy, Low-Calorie Rice Recipes

UNCLE BEN'S, INC.
Houston, Texas 77251

"UNCLE BEN'S," "CONVERTED," and the "PORTRAIT OF UNCLE BEN" are each registered trademarks of UNCLE BEN'S, INC.

Copyright © 1987 by Uncle Ben's, Inc.

All rights reserved. No portion of this book may be reproduced—mechanically, electronically, or by any other means, including photocopying—without written permission from Uncle Ben's, Inc.

Printed in Canada

HOW TO USE THIS BOOK

The book is divided into two sections. The first section includes a one week weight loss plan complete with menus and special diet recipes. The second section features 120 additional low-calorie rice recipes.

THE UNCLE BEN'S 7-DAY RICE DIET®

For the health- and nutrition-conscious consumer who would like to lose weight safely without feeling deprived, the Uncle Ben's 7-Day Rice Diet® can help.

Developed by a registered dietitian in cooperation with the home economists at Uncle Ben's, the diet plan includes a week's worth of nutritionally balanced menus which provide approximately 1,000 calories per day. When combined with a regular exercise program, the Uncle Ben's 7-Day Rice Diet® should result in a gradual weight loss which will vary by individual. Of course, before starting this or any diet, check with your physician.

The plan enables you to enjoy three delicious, satisfying meals each day while working towards a slimmer and healthier you. Each day's menu includes a variety of foods from the four food groups, and limits those which are high in fat, cholesterol and sodium. The diet emphasizes rice which is high in complex carbohydrates. Complex carbohydrate foods tend to be more satisfying. Because you feel less hungry between meals, you're less likely to snack.

The 13 recipes which are part of the Uncle Ben's 7-Day Rice Diet® conform to the strict nutritional parameters of the diet. Therefore, the other 120 recipes in the book *cannot* be substituted in the diet plan. The recipes in the diet plan, however, may be enjoyed anytime.

EASY, LOW-CALORIE RICE RECIPES

If you're not trying to lose weight but would like to improve your eating habits by watching calories and cutting down on fat and sodium, there are 120 additional healthy eating recipes from which to choose. Hearty main dishes, light accompaniment and main dish salads, terrific side dishes, and tempting desserts promise to please everyone's taste.

Streamlined preparation techniques make these recipes extra-convenient. Many are ready to eat in less than 30 minutes; others can be made ahead.

Each recipe includes calorie, protein, carbohydrate, fat and sodium content per serving. These figures, however, should be considered approximate due to the natural variations in the nutritional content of food.

Ingredients listed as optional, unless otherwise stated, are reflected in the nutrition information. If an ingredient is listed with one or more alternatives, such as "1 halibut, haddock or snapper fillet," the first ingredient listed was used to calculate the nutritional content. Thus, in the example just cited, the calculations were based on *1 halibut fillet*. When a range is given for an ingredient, the smaller size or amount was used. For example, in a recipe that calls for "1 can (14½ or 16 ounces) whole tomatoes," the *14½ ounce can* was used. When "salad greens, as desired," appears as a serving or garnish suggestion, ½ cup of iceberg lettuce per serving was used.

All of the recipes in this book were developed to combine the best of both worlds: they're healthful and rich in both flavor and texture. See for yourself how smart eating can be great eating!

The Uncle Ben's 7◊Day Rice Diet®

You've done it! You have decided to shed those unwanted pounds, and now you're wondering just where to start. You know that fad diets can be downright unhealthy, and you dread counting calories and giving up all your favorite foods. The fact is, each day you can eat three delicious, satisfying meals while working towards a slimmer and healthier you with the Uncle Ben's 7-Day Rice Diet®.

Developed by a registered dietitian and nutritionist* in cooperation with home economists at Uncle Ben's, the Uncle Ben's 7-Day Rice Diet® features menu plans and recipes for a week. Each day's menus are nutritionally balanced and provide about 1,000 calories. When combined with a regular exercise program, the 7-Day Menu Plans should result in a gradual weight loss that will vary by individual.

The Uncle Ben's 7-Day Rice Diet® is designed for normal, healthy adults. But before beginning any diet or exercise program, you should check with your physician. A multiple vitamin that meets the U.S. Recommended Dietary Allowances also is recommended due to the low caloric level of the diet.

The Uncle Ben's 7-Day Rice Diet® includes a variety of foods from each of the four basic food groups. It limits foods that are high in fat, cholesterol and sodium and emphasizes UNCLE BEN'S® CONVERTED® Brand Rice, which is fat-free, cholesterol-free and sodium-free.

Rice is a complex carbohydrate food. Complex carbohydrates can be a dieter's best friend. That's because foods which are high in complex carbohydrates tend to be more satisfying. Because you feel less hungry between meals, you are less likely to snack.

---

*Betty Wedman, M.S., R.D., is a nutritionist with an office at the University of Missouri—Columbia. She is a Registered Dietitian and professional member of the American Dietetic Association and American Diabetes Association.

The Uncle Ben's 7-Day Rice Diet® features rice twice a day. You'll be surprised at the many ways in which it is prepared throughout the week. On Tuesday, cooked rice topped with fresh fruit and skim milk gets you going and keeps you going all morning. For Thursday's lunch, tote Chicken Rice Salad Olé and dine at your desk. In the evening, feast on Curried Orange Chicken. All are light and lean yet totally satisfying—for a dieting twosome or a dieter and non-dieting companion.

Streamlined preparation makes the Uncle Ben's 7-Day Rice Diet® convenient, too. Because the recipes and menus have been carefully coordinated, you can prepare enough rice at one time to use in several recipes. One cup of UNCLE BEN'S® CONVERTED® Brand Rice yields over 3 cups of cooked rice—more than enough for three meals. Simply store the cooked rice tightly covered in the refrigerator. Unlike ordinary white rice which can become sticky when chilled and reheated, CONVERTED® Brand Rice retains its separate-grained texture and freshly-prepared flavor.

CONVERTED® Brand Rice also contains more natural rice nutrients. The special processing method which removes the excess surface starch forces vitamins and minerals contained in the outer bran layer toward the center of the rice grain. As a result, after milling, UNCLE BEN'S® contains twice the amount of natural B-complex vitamins as ordinary rice.

The recipes may be enjoyed anytime. They use "light" preparation techniques and lots of fresh, healthy ingredients. Herbs, spices and lemon juice, for example, are often used as replacements for salt.

Rice Diet

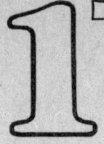

MONDAY MENU

BREAKFAST

½ cup orange juice
1 bran muffin
1 tsp. margarine

LUNCH

1 serving Oriental Tuna Rice Salad*
1 medium apple

DINNER

1 serving Curried Orange Chicken*
½ cup cooked peas and carrots
1 serving tossed vegetable salad with
2 Tbsp. low-calorie dressing

Monday: 1,047 calories, 65 g protein,
25 g fat, 142 g carbohydrate,
1,949 mg sodium

*Recipe included. (Coffee, tea or diet soft drinks are optional beverages.)

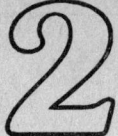

TUESDAY MENU

BREAKFAST

½ cup cooked UNCLE BEN'S® CONVERTED® Brand Rice
½ banana, sliced
½ cup skim milk

LUNCH

1 turkey sandwich (2 slices whole wheat bread, 2 oz. light meat turkey, 1 tsp. mayonnaise, 2 lettuce leaves)
12 grapes

DINNER

1 serving Lemon Veal Chops with Herbed Rice*
2 steamed broccoli spears
1 cup strawberries

Tuesday: 944 calories, 57 g protein, 20 g fat, 134 g carbohydrate, 1,370 mg sodium

*Recipe included. (Coffee, tea or diet soft drinks are optional beverages.)

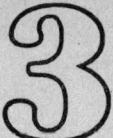

WEDNESDAY MENU

BREAKFAST

½ cup blueberries
¾ cup corn flakes
½ cup skim milk

LUNCH

1 serving Manhattan Style Fish Chowder*
1 serving tossed vegetable salad with
2 Tbsp. low-calorie dressing

DINNER

Baked chicken breast half
1 serving Slim Spanish Rice*
1 cup fresh fruit
½ cup plain low-fat yogurt

*Wednesday: 1,004 calories, 68 g protein,
12 g fat, 156 g carbohydrate,
1,908 mg sodium*

*Recipe included. (Coffee, tea or diet soft drinks are optional beverages.)

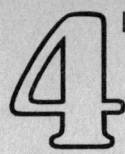

THURSDAY MENU

BREAKFAST

½ grapefruit
¼ cup cottage cheese on
1 slice whole wheat toast

LUNCH

1 serving Chicken Rice Salad Olé*
3 soda crackers

DINNER

1 serving Gingered Pork and Pea Pods*
1 medium pear

*Thursday: 992 calories, 61 g protein,
37 g fat, 103 g carbohydrate,
1,773 mg sodium*

*Recipe included. (Coffee, tea or diet soft drinks are optional beverages.)

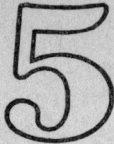

FRIDAY MENU

BREAKFAST

1 English muffin
1 Tbsp. peanut butter

LUNCH

1 serving Three Fruit Rice Salad*
½ cup cottage cheese

DINNER

1 serving South of the Border Shrimpy Rice*
½ cup steamed green beans

Friday: 939 calories, 54 g protein, 26 g fat, 119 g carbohydrate, 1,535 mg sodium

*Recipe included. (Coffee, tea or diet soft drinks are optional beverages.)

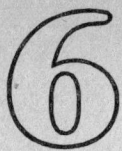

SATURDAY MENU

BREAKFAST

4 prunes
1 poached egg
1 slice whole wheat toast
1 tsp. margarine

LUNCH

1 serving Vegetarian Rice Bake*
1 medium peach

DINNER

Baked Cornish Hen half
1 serving Quick 'n Easy Ratatouille Rice*
4 steamed asparagus spears
1 serving romaine lettuce salad with
2 Tbsp. low-calorie dressing

Saturday: 1,008 calories, 58 g protein, 21 g fat, 145 g carbohydrate, 1,675 mg sodium

*Recipe included. (Coffee, tea or diet soft drinks are optional beverages.)

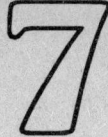

SUNDAY MENU

BRUNCH

1 serving Fisherman's Frittata*
½ cantaloupe

DINNER

1 cup vegetable soup
2 oz. low-fat mozzarella cheese
3 Rye-Crisp
1 serving Mexican Chocolate Rice Cream*

Sunday: 1,030 calories, 72 g protein, 29 g fat, 118 g carbohydrate, 2,490 mg sodium

*Recipe included. (Coffee, tea or diet soft drinks are optional beverages.)

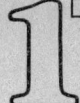

MONDAY RECIPES

ORIENTAL TUNA RICE SALAD

2½ cups water
1 cup UNCLE BEN'S® CONVERTED® Brand Rice
3 tablespoons red wine vinegar
1½ tablespoons vegetable oil
2 to 3 teaspoons soy sauce
½ to ¾ teaspoon grated fresh ginger
1 can (6½ ounces) tuna, packed in water, drained
½ cup fresh bean sprouts
½ cup sliced celery
¼ cup thinly sliced radishes
1 cup shredded fresh spinach

Prepare rice according to package directions. Reserve 1 cup in medium bowl; cool to room temperature. Cover and refrigerate remaining rice.

Combine vinegar, oil, soy sauce and ginger in small bowl. Add to reserved rice with tuna, bean sprouts, celery and radishes; mix well. Cover and chill. Stir in spinach.

Makes 2 servings

Per Serving: *315 calories, 30 g protein, 11 g fat, 23 g carbohydrate, 58 mg cholesterol, 794 mg sodium when prepared with 2 teaspoons soy sauce*

CURRIED ORANGE CHICKEN

- ¾ to 1¼ teaspoons curry powder
- ½ teaspoon salt
- Dash pepper
- 2 chicken breast halves, boned and skinned
- ⅔ cup orange juice
- ⅔ cup water
- ½ cup UNCLE BEN'S® CONVERTED® Brand Rice
- 1 teaspoon brown sugar
- ½ teaspoon dry mustard
- 1 tablespoon chopped parsley

Combine curry powder, ¼ teaspoon of the salt and the pepper. Rub seasonings onto top and bottom surfaces of each chicken piece; set aside. Combine remaining ingredients except parsley in 8-inch skillet; mix well. Bring to a boil. Arrange chicken over rice. Cover tightly and simmer 20 minutes. Remove from heat. Let stand covered until all liquid is absorbed, about 5 minutes. Sprinkle with parsley.

Makes 2 servings

Per Serving: *335 calories, 28 g protein, 3 g fat, 49 g carbohydrate, 59 mg cholesterol, 587 mg sodium*

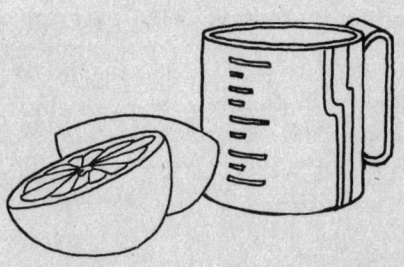

2 TUESDAY RECIPE

LEMON VEAL CHOPS WITH HERBED RICE

- 1⅓ cups + 3 tablespoons water
- 1¼ teaspoons chicken bouillon granules
- ½ cup UNCLE BEN'S® CONVERTED® Brand Rice
- ⅔ cup coarsely chopped onion
- 2 garlic cloves, minced
- ½ teaspoon each: basil, oregano
- 2 veal chops, 4 ounces each (about ½ inch thick)
- ¼ teaspoon salt
- Dash cayenne pepper
- 3 tablespoons dry white wine
- ½ lemon, thinly sliced
- 2 teaspoons chopped parsley
- Freshly ground pepper, to taste

Bring 1⅓ cups water and 1 teaspoon of the bouillon granules to a boil in small saucepan. Stir in the next 5 ingredients. Cover tightly and simmer 20 minutes. While rice cooks, season veal chops with salt and cayenne pepper. Heat 8-inch non-stick skillet over medium heat until hot. Sear chops on both sides. Reduce heat. Add remaining 3 tablespoons water, wine and remaining ¼ teaspoon bouillon granules. Arrange lemon slices on top of chops. Cover and cook over low heat until veal is tender, about 15 minutes. Remove rice from heat. Let stand covered until all liquid is absorbed, about 5 minutes. Stir in parsley and pepper. Serve with veal chops, spooning juices over chops.   *Makes 2 servings*

Per Serving: 375 calories, 23 g protein, 11 g fat, 45 g carbohydrate, 68 mg cholesterol, 642 mg sodium

3 WEDNESDAY RECIPES

MANHATTAN STYLE FISH CHOWDER

- 2 cups vegetable juice cocktail
- 1 large tomato, coarsely chopped
- ½ cup coarsely chopped onion
- 1 small green pepper, cut into ¾-inch pieces
- 2 garlic cloves, minced
- 1 teaspoon lemon juice
- ½ teaspoon basil, crushed
- ¼ teaspoon oregano, crushed
- 1 cup cooked UNCLE BEN'S® CONVERTED® Brand Rice
- ½ pound sole, flounder or haddock fillets, cut into bite-size pieces
- Freshly ground pepper, to taste

Combine first 8 ingredients in medium saucepan. Bring to a boil. Reduce heat. Cover and simmer 15 minutes, stirring occasionally. Add rice and fish. Continue cooking until fish flakes easily with fork, about 5 minutes. Sprinkle with pepper.

Makes 2 servings

Per Serving: 245 calories, 23 g protein, 1 g fat, 36 g carbohydrate, 60 mg cholesterol, 819 mg sodium

SLIM SPANISH RICE

1 can (8 ounces) whole tomatoes (1 cup)
½ cup UNCLE BEN'S® CONVERTED® Brand Rice
⅓ cup chopped onion
¼ cup chopped green pepper
¼ cup thinly sliced celery
1 small bay leaf
1 garlic clove, minced
⅛ to ¼ teaspoon dried red pepper flakes
¼ teaspoon each: thyme, salt

Drain and coarsely chop tomatoes, reserving juice. Add enough water to juice to equal 1⅓ cups. Bring to a boil in small saucepan. Stir in remaining ingredients including tomatoes. Cover tightly and simmer 20 minutes. Remove from heat. Let stand covered until most of liquid is absorbed, about 5 minutes. Remove bay leaf.

Makes 2 servings

Per Serving: *212 calories, 5 g protein, less than 1 g fat, 47 g carbohydrate, 0 mg cholesterol, 442 mg sodium*

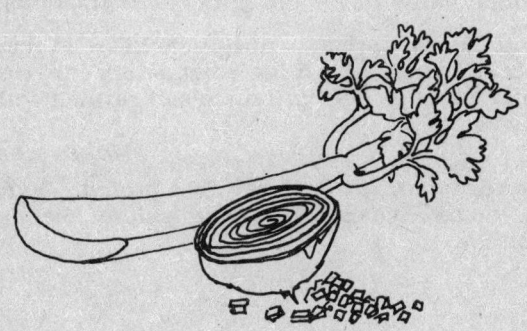

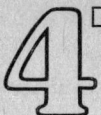

THURSDAY RECIPES

CHICKEN RICE SALAD OLÉ

2½ cups water
1 cup UNCLE BEN'S® CONVERTED® Brand Rice
1 cup diced cooked chicken
½ cup green pepper strips
1 to 2 tablespoons canned chopped green chilies, drained
⅓ cup plain low-fat yogurt
2 teaspoons cider vinegar
¼ teaspoon each: salt, cumin, chili powder
1 small tomato, coarsely chopped
1 tablespoon sliced pitted ripe olives

Prepare rice according to package directions. Reserve 1 cup in medium bowl; cool to room temperature. Cover and refrigerate remaining rice.

Add chicken, green pepper and chilies to reserved rice. Combine next 5 ingredients. Stir into rice mixture; chill. Stir in tomato and garnish with olives.

Makes 2 servings

Per Serving: *235 calories, 26 g protein, 4 g fat, 23 g carbohydrate, 58 mg cholesterol, 641 mg sodium*

GINGERED PORK AND PEA PODS

- 2 teaspoons soy sauce
- ¾ teaspoon grated fresh ginger
- ¼ teaspoon dried red pepper flakes
- ½ pound lean pork loin, cut into thin bite-size strips
- 2 garlic cloves, minced
- 1 cup cooked UNCLE BEN'S® CONVERTED® Brand Rice
- ½ cup red pepper strips
- 3 ounces frozen pea pods, thawed and drained
- 2 tablespoons thinly sliced green onion

Combine first 3 ingredients; set aside. Heat large non-stick skillet over medium heat until hot. Add pork strips; stir-fry 2 minutes. Add garlic; stir-fry 1 to 2 minutes or until pork is no longer pink. Add rice; stir-fry 2 to 3 minutes. Add red pepper strips, pea pods, onion and soy sauce mixture; stir-fry 3 minutes or until hot.

Makes 2 servings

Per Serving: *450 calories, 23 g protein, 29 g fat, 24 g carbohydrate, 70 mg cholesterol, 773 mg sodium*

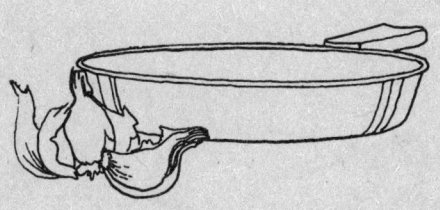

5 FRIDAY RECIPES

THREE FRUIT RICE SALAD

3 tablespoons orange juice
1½ tablespoons vegetable oil
1 teaspoon lemon juice
1 teaspoon sugar
¾ teaspoon chopped fresh mint leaves
  OR ¼ teaspoon dried mint
½ teaspoon each: poppy seeds, grated orange peel
1 cup cooked UNCLE BEN'S® CONVERTED® Brand Rice
¾ cup small cantaloupe balls
½ cup each: sliced strawberries, pineapple chunks

Combine first 4 ingredients. Add mint, poppy seeds and orange peel; mix well. Stir dressing into rice. Cover and chill several hours. Stir in fruits.

Makes 2 servings

Per Serving: *240 calories, 2 g protein, 10 g fat, 35 g carbohydrate, 0 mg cholesterol, 268 mg sodium*

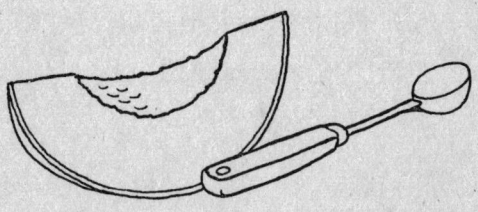

SOUTH OF THE BORDER SHRIMPY RICE

1 can (8 ounces) whole tomatoes (1 cup)
⅓ cup coarsely chopped onion
1 large garlic clove, minced
½ cup UNCLE BEN'S® CONVERTED® Brand Rice
1 bay leaf
10 small pimiento-stuffed green olives
½ pound medium frozen cooked shrimp, thawed
1 small green pepper, cut into thin strips

Drain and chop tomatoes, reserving juice. Add enough water to juice to equal 1⅓ cups. Combine tomatoes, tomato liquid, onion and garlic in 8-inch skillet. Bring to a boil. Stir in rice, bay leaf and olives. Cover tightly and simmer 20 minutes. Stir in shrimp and green pepper. Remove from heat. Let stand covered until all liquid is absorbed, about 5 minutes. Remove bay leaf.

Makes 2 servings

Per Serving: *340 calories, 29 g protein, 3 g fat, 49 g carbohydrate, 199 mg cholesterol, 677 mg sodium*

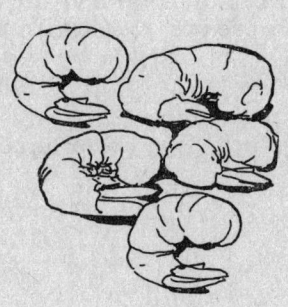

6 SATURDAY RECIPES

VEGETARIAN RICE BAKE

1 can (8 ounces) whole tomatoes (1 cup)
1 can (8¾ ounces) kidney beans, drained (¾ cup drained)
½ cup UNCLE BEN'S® CONVERTED® Brand Rice
⅔ cup sliced zucchini
½ cup chopped onion
1 teaspoon chili powder
¾ teaspoon cumin
¼ teaspoon garlic salt
¼ cup green pepper strips
¼ cup (1 ounce) shredded low-moisture, part-skim mozzarella cheese

Drain and chop tomatoes, reserving juice. Add enough water to juice to equal 1⅓ cups. Combine tomatoes, tomato liquid, and next 7 ingredients in 8-inch square baking dish; mix well. Cover tightly with foil. Bake at 350°F. 45 minutes or until most of liquid is absorbed. Uncover and stir. Sprinkle green pepper and cheese over top. Return to oven to melt cheese.

Makes 2 servings

Per Serving: 343 calories, 15 g protein, 3 g fat, 64 g carbohydrate, 8 mg cholesterol, 501 mg sodium

QUICK 'N EASY RATATOUILLE RICE

2½ cups water
1 cup UNCLE BEN'S® CONVERTED® Brand Rice
⅔ cup chopped onion
⅓ cup sliced yellow squash
⅓ cup sliced zucchini
¼ cup coarsely chopped red or green pepper
1 garlic clove, minced
1 teaspoon basil
¼ teaspoon salt
1 small tomato, diced
2 teaspoons chopped parsley

Prepare rice according to package directions. Reserve 1 cup. Cover and refrigerate remaining rice.

Cook onion in 8-inch non-stick skillet, stirring constantly, 1 minute. Stir in the next 6 ingredients. Cover and cook over low heat, stirring occasionally, until vegetables are tender, about 10 minutes. Stir in tomato and reserved rice. Cook, covered, 10 minutes longer, stirring several times. Sprinkle with parsley.

Makes 2 servings

Per Serving: *118 calories, 3 g protein, less than 1 g fat, 26 g carbohydrate, 0 mg cholesterol, 535 mg sodium*

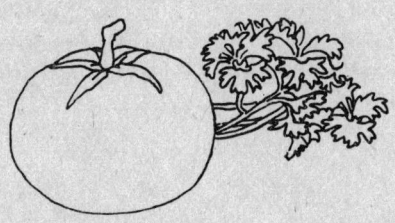

7 SUNDAY RECIPES

FISHERMAN'S FRITTATA

3 large eggs
1 cup cooked UNCLE BEN'S® CONVERTED® Brand Rice
1 can (6½ ounces) tuna, packed in water, drained and flaked
½ cup diced red pepper
2 tablespoons thinly sliced green onion
¼ teaspoon garlic salt
Dash pepper
2 teaspoons margarine
¼ cup (1 ounce) shredded low-moisture, part-skim mozzarella cheese
1 tablespoon grated Parmesan cheese

Beat eggs thoroughly. Stir in remaining ingredients except margarine and cheeses; mix well. Melt margarine in 8-inch non-stick skillet over medium-high heat until bubbly but not brown. Pour in egg mixture; cover. Reduce heat to low. Cook until eggs are set and edges are puffy, about 15 minutes. Sprinkle with cheeses.

Makes 2 servings

Per Serving: *400 calories, 42 g protein, 16 g fat, 21 g carbohydrate, 448 mg cholesterol, 800 mg sodium*

MEXICAN CHOCOLATE RICE CREAM

 3 tablespoons sugar
 1½ tablespoons unsweetened cocoa
 2½ teaspoons cornstarch
 1 cup skim milk
 1 cup cooked UNCLE BEN'S® CONVERTED® Brand Rice
 ¾ teaspoon vanilla
 Ground cinnamon, as desired

Combine first 3 ingredients in small saucepan. Gradually stir in milk. Cook over medium heat, stirring constantly, until mixture comes to a boil. Boil 1 minute, stirring constantly. Remove from heat. Stir in rice and vanilla. Spoon into serving dishes. Serve warm or chilled, sprinkled with cinnamon.

Makes 2 servings

***Per Serving:** 215 calories, 6 g protein, less than 1 g fat, 46 g carbohydrate, 3 mg cholesterol, 324 mg sodium*

Nutrition Information for UNCLE BEN'S® CONVERTED® Brand Rice

SERVING SIZE . . ½ Cup
Per Serving
Calories 100
Protein, g 2
Carbohydrate, g 22
Fat, g 0
Sodium, mg 0

Percentage of U.S. Recommended Daily Allowance (U.S. RDA) Per Serving
Protein 2
Vitamin A . . . . *
Vitamin C . . . . *
Thiamine 8
Riboflavin . . . . *
Niacin 4
Calcium . . . . *
Iron 4

*Contains less than 2 percent of U.S. RDA of these nutrients

Main Dishes

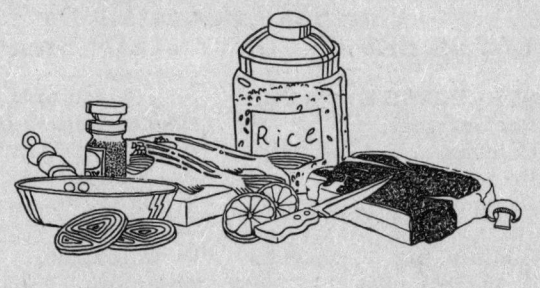

CHICKEN WITH PIMIENTO SAUCE OVER GREEN RICE

1 can (13¾ or 14½ ounces) chicken broth
1 cup UNCLE BEN'S® CONVERTED® Brand Rice
1 jar (4 ounces) whole pimientos
¾ cup dry white wine
1 teaspoon sugar
½ teaspoon dried basil, crushed
Salt and pepper, to taste
6 chicken breast halves, boned and skinned
1 tablespoon margarine
2 tablespoons plain low-fat yogurt
3 tablespoons chopped parsley
3 tablespoons chopped chives

Add enough water to chicken broth to equal 2½ cups. Bring to a boil in medium saucepan. Stir in rice. Cover tightly and simmer 20 minutes. While rice is cooking, combine pimientos including liquid, wine, sugar and basil in blender container; blend until smooth. Salt and pepper chicken breast halves. Cook chicken in margarine in 12-inch non-stick skillet over medium heat until firm and cooked through, about 7 minutes on each side. Remove chicken from skillet; keep warm. Add pimiento mixture to skillet. Cook over medium-high heat, stirring occasionally, until slightly thickened, about 10 minutes. Stir in yogurt; heat through but do not boil. Remove rice from heat. Let stand covered until all liquid is absorbed, about 5 minutes. Stir in parsley and chives. Arrange chicken and rice on serving platter. Serve with pimiento sauce.

Makes 6 servings

Per Serving: *300 calories, 31 g protein, 4 g fat, 29 g carbohydrate, 313 mg sodium when prepared without salt*

PACIFIC PAELLA

- 4 chicken breast halves, boned and skinned
- 1 teaspoon paprika
- 1 teaspoon salt (optional)
- ¼ teaspoon pepper
- ½ pound mild Italian sausage
- 1 can (14½ or 16 ounces) whole tomatoes
- 2 cans (13¾ or 14½ ounces each) chicken broth
- ½ teaspoon turmeric
- ¼ teaspoon saffron (optional)
- 2 cups UNCLE BEN'S® CONVERTED® Brand Rice
- 1 large onion, cut into wedges
- 2 garlic cloves, minced
- 1 pound medium shrimp, peeled, deveined and cooked
- 1 green pepper, cut into thin strips
- 10 mussels, cleaned and steamed (optional)

Cut chicken breasts into ½-inch strips. Combine paprika, salt, if desired, and pepper in small bowl. Add chicken and stir until all seasoning is worked into chicken. Cut sausage into ¼-inch pieces; remove casing. Drain and coarsely chop tomatoes, reserving liquid for another use. Add enough water to chicken broth to make 3¾ cups. Bring to a boil in 12-inch skillet. Stir in turmeric, saffron, rice, onion, garlic, chicken, sausage and tomatoes. Cover tightly and simmer 20 minutes. Remove from heat. Stir in shrimp and green pepper; if desired, top with mussels. Let stand covered until all liquid is absorbed, about 5 minutes.

Makes 10 servings

Per Serving: *345 calories, 30 g protein, 9 g fat, 35 g carbohydrate, 772 mg sodium when prepared with salt and saffron, but without mussels*

FISH AND RICE MARINARA

- 1 package (16 ounces) frozen cod, flounder or sole fillets
- 1 tablespoon lemon juice
- 1 can (14½ ounces) stewed tomatoes
- 1 cup dry white wine
- 1½ teaspoons dried basil, crushed
- 1½ teaspoons onion salt
- ¾ teaspoon dried oregano, crushed
- ⅛ teaspoon pepper
- 1 cup UNCLE BEN'S® CONVERTED® Brand Rice
- 1 large carrot, cut into ¼-inch thick slices
- 1 large green pepper, cut into thin strips
- Paprika

Let frozen fish stand at room temperature 20 to 30 minutes to thaw slightly. Cut block of fish lengthwise in half, then crosswise into 16 pieces. Drizzle with lemon juice and set aside. Combine tomatoes, wine, basil, onion salt, oregano and pepper in 10-inch skillet. Bring to a boil. Stir in rice, carrot and fish. Cover tightly and simmer 20 minutes. Arrange green pepper strips on top of rice mixture. Remove from heat. Let stand covered until all liquid is absorbed, about 5 minutes. Sprinkle with paprika.

Makes 6 servings

Per Serving: *285 calories, 19 g protein, 7 g fat, 35 g carbohydrate, 686 mg sodium*

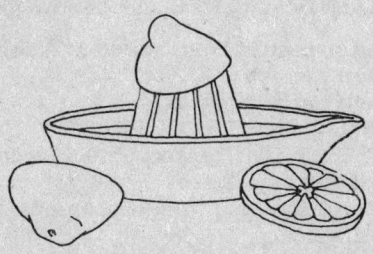

Main Dishes 33

LEMON FISH AND RICE AMANDINE

2¼ cups water
¼ cup lemon juice
1 cup UNCLE BEN'S® CONVERTED® Brand Rice
1 teaspoon salt
⅛ teaspoon ground nutmeg
¼ cup sliced green onions with tops
1 package (16 ounces) frozen cod, flounder or sole fillets, thawed, cut into 6 serving pieces
Paprika
1½ tablespoons margarine, melted
1 lemon, thinly sliced
2 tablespoons sliced almonds

Bring water and lemon juice to a boil in medium saucepan. Stir in rice, salt and nutmeg. Cover tightly and simmer 20 minutes. Remove from heat. Let stand covered until all liquid is absorbed, about 5 minutes. Stir in green onions. Spoon rice into 13×9×2-inch baking dish. Arrange fish over rice; sprinkle lightly with paprika. Drizzle fish with margarine; top with lemon slices and sprinkle with almonds. Cover loosely with aluminum foil. Bake at 400°F. 12 to 15 minutes or until fish flakes when tested with a fork.

Makes 6 servings

Per Serving: 225 calories, 16 g protein, 5 g fat, 28 g carbohydrate, 445 mg sodium

CANTONESE CHICKEN AND RICE

6 chicken breast halves, boned and skinned
¼ teaspoon pepper
⅛ teaspoon garlic powder
1 cup UNCLE BEN'S® CONVERTED® Brand Rice
1 can (13¾ or 14½ ounces) chicken broth
3 tablespoons soy sauce
1 package (6 ounces) frozen pea pods, thawed and drained
1 jar (2 ounces) sliced pimiento, drained

Sprinkle chicken with pepper and garlic powder. Combine rice, chicken broth and 2 tablespoons of the soy sauce in 10-inch skillet. Arrange chicken over rice. Bring to a boil. Reduce heat. Cover tightly and simmer 20 minutes. Uncover and spoon remaining 1 tablespoon soy sauce over chicken. Top with pea pods and pimiento. Remove from heat. Let stand covered until all liquid is absorbed, about 5 minutes.

Makes 6 servings

Per Serving: 270 calories, 32 g protein, 2 g fat, 29 g carbohydrate, 801 mg sodium

SPRING GARDEN BROWN RICE SUPPER

1 garlic clove, minced
2 teaspoons margarine
2⅔ cups water
1 teaspoon salt (optional)
¼ teaspoon ground nutmeg
1 cup UNCLE BEN'S® Select Brown Rice
2 cups small broccoli flowerets
½ pound mushrooms, thinly sliced
1 cup cherry tomatoes, halved
¾ cup (3 ounces) shredded low-moisture, part-skim mozzarella cheese

Cook garlic in margarine in 10-inch non-stick skillet 2 minutes. Add water, salt, if desired, and nutmeg; bring to a boil. Stir in rice. Cover tightly and cook over low heat 40 minutes. Top with broccoli. Cover and continue cooking over low heat until all liquid is absorbed, about 10 minutes. Stir in mushrooms and tomatoes; heat through. Sprinkle with cheese.

Makes 4 servings

Per Serving: 295 calories, 13 g protein, 7 g fat, 44 g carbohydrate, 690 mg sodium when prepared with salt

SCALLOP STIR FRY

1 can (8 ounces) pineapple chunks, packed in juice
1 pound bay scallops, rinsed and drained
2 medium carrots, cut into matchstick strips
½ cup sliced green onions with tops
1 garlic clove, minced
1 tablespoon vegetable oil
⅓ cup chicken broth
2 tablespoons reduced sodium soy sauce
½ teaspoon ground ginger
¼ teaspoon pepper
1 tablespoon cornstarch
2 cups snow peas, trimmed*
3 cups hot cooked rice**

Drain pineapple, reserving juice. Cut pineapple chunks in half. Stir-fry pineapple, scallops, carrots, onions and garlic in oil in wok or large skillet 2 to 3 minutes. Combine chicken broth, soy sauce, 2 tablespoons of the reserved pineapple juice, ginger and pepper. Add to cornstarch, stirring until smooth. Add to wok with snow peas. Cook, stirring constantly, until sauce is clear and thickened, 2 to 3 minutes. Serve over rice.

Makes 6 servings

*One package (6 ounces) frozen pea pods, thawed and drained, may be substituted.

**Prepared without butter or salt.

Per Serving: 220 calories, 14 g protein, 3 g fat, 30 g carbohydrate, 435 mg sodium

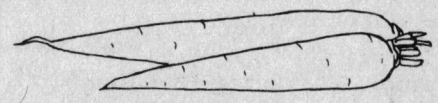

BEEF & SNOW PEAS CHINESE-STYLE

- ¾ pound boneless beef top round steak
- 2 tablespoons cornstarch
- 2 tablespoons soy sauce
- 1 tablespoon dry sherry
- ½ teaspoon sugar
- ½ teaspoon salt
- 1 cup UNCLE BEN'S® CONVERTED® Brand Rice
- 1 tablespoon vegetable oil
- ¾ cup water
- 1 can (8 ounces) water chestnuts, drained and sliced
- 1 package (6 ounces) frozen pea pods, thawed
- 2 tablespoons chopped green onions with tops
- 2 tablespoons pimiento strips

Trim meat of all visible fat; chill in freezer until slightly firm. Cut meat diagonally across the grain into very thin slices; place in shallow baking dish. Combine 1 tablespoon of the cornstarch, the soy sauce, sherry, sugar and salt; pour over meat. Let stand 30 minutes. Prepare rice according to package directions omitting butter. Drain beef, reserving marinade. Heat oil in large non-stick skillet until hot but not smoking. Add beef to skillet. Cook and stir until browned, 3 to 4 minutes. Combine remaining 1 tablespoon cornstarch and the water with meat marinade; mix well. Add to skillet with water chestnuts and pea pods. Cook and stir until sauce is thickened and clear. Stir green onions and pimiento into rice. Serve meat mixture over rice.

Makes 6 servings

Per Serving: *300 calories, 14 g protein, 10 g fat, 35 g carbohydrate, 916 mg sodium*

MIXED VEGETABLE CURRY AND SPICY RICE

- 3½ cups water
- 1 cup UNCLE BEN'S® CONVERTED® Brand Rice
- 1 tablespoon margarine
- 3 carrots, sliced diagonally
- 1 medium onion, sliced
- 1 garlic clove
- 1½ teaspoons ground coriander
- 1 teaspoon turmeric
- ½ teaspoon ground ginger
- ⅛ teaspoon cayenne pepper
- 1 small head cauliflower (about 1 pound), broken into flowerets
- 2 teaspoons cornstarch
- 1 teaspoon salt (optional)
- ¼ cup chopped walnuts
- ¼ cup raisins
- ¼ teaspoon ground cinnamon
- ⅛ teaspoon ground cloves

Bring 2½ cups of the water to a boil in medium saucepan. Stir in rice. Cover tightly and simmer 20 minutes. While rice is cooking, melt margarine in large saucepan. Add carrots, onion and garlic. Cook over medium heat, stirring occasionally, 2 to 3 minutes. Stir in coriander, turmeric, ginger, cayenne pepper and ½ cup of the water. Cover tightly and cook over low heat about 10 minutes. Add cauliflower. Cover and continue cooking until vegetables are tender, about 10 minutes. Combine remaining ½ cup water, cornstarch and, if desired, salt. Stir until smooth. Add to vegetables. Cook, stirring constantly, until thickened. Remove rice from heat. Stir in remaining ingredients. Let stand covered until all liquid is absorbed, about 5 minutes. Serve curry over rice.   *Makes 6 servings*

Per Serving: 240 calories, 6 g protein, 5 g fat, 42 g carbohydrate, 411 mg sodium when prepared with salt

GYPSY FRIED RICE

¾ pound beef chuck, trimmed of visible fat and
    cut into small cubes
1 tablespoon margarine
1 small onion, chopped
2 large carrots, sliced
2 medium green peppers OR 1 red and 1 green
    pepper, cut into thin strips
⅔ cup dry white wine
1 bay leaf
1 teaspoon salt
Dash pepper
2½ cups beef broth or bouillon
1 cup UNCLE BEN'S® CONVERTED® Brand Rice
1 cup plain low-fat yogurt

Cook beef in margarine in large non-stick skillet over medium heat until lightly browned. Add onion, carrots and peppers. Cook, stirring occasionally, until onion is tender. Add wine, bay leaf, salt and pepper. Cover tightly and simmer until meat is tender, about 1 hour. While meat is cooking, bring broth to a boil in medium saucepan. Stir in rice. Cover tightly and simmer 20 minutes. Remove from heat. Let stand covered until all liquid is absorbed, about 5 minutes. Remove bay leaf from meat mixture. Add hot cooked rice; mix well. Remove from heat. Stir in yogurt.

Makes 6 servings

Per Serving: *325 calories, 17 g protein, 11 g fat, 35 g carbohydrate, 786 mg sodium*

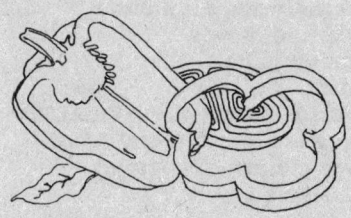

Main Dishes 39

CIOPPINO RICE SKILLET

1¼ cups tomato juice
¾ cup water
½ cup UNCLE BEN'S® CONVERTED® Brand Rice
⅓ cup coarsely chopped onion
2 garlic cloves, minced
1 teaspoon dried basil, crushed
¾ teaspoon dried oregano, crushed
1 halibut, haddock or snapper fillet, ½ to ¾ inch thick (about ¼ pound), cut in half
¼ pound cooked and cleaned medium shrimp
1 can (6½ ounces) minced clams, drained
1 small green pepper, cut into matchstick strips
Paprika
Lemon wedges

Bring tomato juice and water to a boil in 10-inch skillet. Stir in rice, onion, garlic, basil and oregano. Arrange fish on top. Cover tightly and simmer 20 minutes. Gently stir in shrimp, clams and green pepper. Remove from heat. Let stand covered until all liquid is absorbed, about 5 minutes. Sprinkle fish with paprika. Serve with lemon wedges.

Makes 2 servings

Per Serving: 390 calories, 39 g protein, 2 g fat, 53 g carbohydrate, 483 mg sodium

CHICKEN AND RICE MONTEREY

2 chicken breast halves, boned and skinned
½ teaspoon salt
⅛ teaspoon ground cinnamon
Dash ground cloves
⅔ cup orange juice
⅔ cup water
½ cup UNCLE BEN'S® CONVERTED® Brand Rice
1 small tomato, seeded and diced
Chopped cilantro or parsley
Orange slices

Cut chicken breasts into 2×½×½-inch strips. Combine salt, cinnamon and cloves in bowl. Add chicken strips and stir until all of the seasoning mixture is worked into chicken; set aside. Bring orange juice and water to a boil in medium skillet. Stir in rice, tomato and chicken. Cover tightly and simmer 20 minutes. Remove from heat. Let stand covered until all liquid is absorbed, about 5 minutes. Sprinkle with cilantro and garnish with orange slices.

Makes 2 servings

Per Serving: 340 calories, 28 g protein, 3 g fat, 49 g carbohydrate, 587 mg sodium when prepared without garnishes

MEXICAN TURKEY BAKE

- 1 cup UNCLE BEN'S® CONVERTED® Brand Rice
- 1 can (about 3 ounces) mild green chilies, drained and chopped
- 3 cups cubed cooked turkey
- 1 can (12 ounces) Mexican-style corn with sweet peppers, drained
- 1 can (10 ounces) enchilada sauce
- ¾ teaspoon salt (optional)
- 1 cup plain low-fat yogurt

Prepare rice according to package directions omitting butter. Reserve 1 tablespoon chilies for garnish. Combine remaining chilies, turkey, corn, enchilada sauce, salt, if desired, and cooked rice in large bowl. Spoon into greased 13×9×2-inch baking dish. Cover and bake at 350°F. until hot, about 25 minutes. Spoon yogurt down center and garnish with reserved chilies.

Makes 6 servings

Per Serving: 315 calories, 27 g protein, 4 g fat, 42 g carbohydrate, 1102 mg sodium when prepared with salt

ROSEMARY CHICKEN KABOBS

- 6 chicken breast halves, boned and skinned
- 1 teaspoon paprika
- 1 cup white wine
- 1 tablespoon vegetable oil
- 1 teaspoon dried rosemary, crushed
- 2 garlic cloves, minced
- 2½ cups chicken broth or bouillon
- 1 cup UNCLE BEN'S® CONVERTED® Brand Rice
- 2 medium yellow squash, cut into ½-inch thick slices
- 1 medium zucchini, cut into ½-inch thick slices
- 1 large red or green pepper, cut into 1-inch squares
- 2 tablespoons chopped green onions with tops

Cut chicken into 1½-inch cubes. Add paprika; stir to coat. Combine wine, oil, rosemary and garlic; pour over chicken. Marinate at room temperature one hour. About 30 minutes before serving, bring broth to a boil in medium saucepan. Stir in rice. Cover tightly and simmer 20 minutes. Meanwhile, thread chicken onto skewers alternately with yellow squash, zucchini and pepper. Brush with marinade. Cook under broiler, 4 to 5 inches from heat source, or on grill, about 8 to 10 minutes, until chicken is cooked through. Turn once and baste with marinade during cooking. Remove rice from heat. Let stand covered until all liquid is absorbed, about 5 minutes. Stir in onion. Arrange kabobs over rice.

Makes 6 servings

Per Serving: *310 calories, 32 g protein, 4 g fat, 32 g carbohydrate, 384 mg sodium*

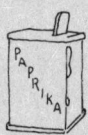

ITALIAN-STYLE FISH AND BROWN RICE BAKE

 1 pound frozen flounder or sole fillets, thawed
 ¼ cup reduced calorie Italian-style salad dressing
 1 teaspoon dried basil, crushed
 ⅔ cup chopped onion
 2 teaspoons margarine
 2⅔ cups water
 1 teaspoon salt (optional)
 1 cup UNCLE BEN'S® Select Brown Rice
 1 package (10 ounces) frozen chopped broccoli, thawed and drained
 1 medium tomato, cut into 6 slices

Combine fish, dressing and basil in plastic bag; seal tightly. Refrigerate while rice is cooking, turning occasionally. Cook onion in margarine in large saucepan until tender but not brown. Add water and, if desired, salt; bring to a boil. Stir in rice. Cover tightly and cook over low heat until all water is absorbed, about 50 minutes. Stir in broccoli. Heat oven to 400°F. Spoon rice mixture into 11×7×2-inch baking dish, forming an even layer. Drain fish, reserving dressing mixture. Arrange fish over rice. Top fish with tomato slices. Drizzle with reserved dressing mixture. Bake uncovered at 400°F. until fish flakes when tested with a fork, about 15 minutes.

Makes 6 servings

Per Serving: *220 calories, 17 g protein, 4 g fat, 29 g carbohydrate, 518 mg sodium when prepared with salt*

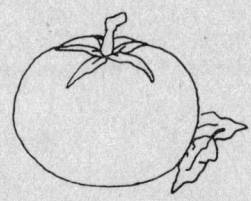

MARINATED SHRIMP KABOBS WITH CONFETTI RICE

- ¼ cup dry sherry
- 1½ teaspoons lemon juice
- 1 garlic clove, crushed
- 1 teaspoon finely minced parsley
- ½ pound jumbo shrimp (16 to 18 per pound), peeled and deveined, with tails left on
- 1 can (8 ounces) pineapple chunks, packed in juice
- ½ cup UNCLE BEN'S® CONVERTED® Brand Rice
- 6 cherry tomatoes, halved
- 2 green onions with tops, thinly sliced
- 2 teaspoons soy sauce
- 1 teaspoon grated fresh ginger, or as desired

Combine sherry, lemon juice, garlic and parsley in shallow container. Add shrimp; mix well. Cover and refrigerate 3 to 4 hours, stirring occasionally.

About 30 minutes before serving, drain pineapple, reserving juice. Add enough water to juice to equal 1⅓ cups; bring to a boil in medium saucepan. Stir in rice. Cover tightly and simmer 20 minutes. Meanwhile, remove shrimp from marinade, reserving marinade. Thread shrimp onto 2 skewers. Brush with marinade. Cook under broiler, 4 to 5 inches from heat source, or on grill, 3 to 4 minutes on each side, or until shrimp are cooked. Brush frequently with marinade. While shrimp are cooking, remove rice from heat. Stir in tomatoes, onion, soy sauce, ginger and pineapple. Let stand covered until all liquid is absorbed, about 5 minutes. Serve kabobs over rice.

Makes 2 servings

Per Serving: *400 calories, 27 g protein, 2 g fat, 68 g carbohydrate, 512 mg sodium*

TARRAGON CHICKEN WITH CALIFORNIA RICE

1⅔ cups water
1 cup chicken broth
1 cup UNCLE BEN'S® Select Brown Rice
1 teaspoon dried tarragon, crushed
½ teaspoon salt
¼ teaspoon pepper
6 chicken breast halves, boned and skinned
1 tablespoon margarine
¼ cup red or green pepper strips
3 tablespoons slivered almonds
1 tablespoon finely chopped green onions with tops

Bring water and chicken broth to a boil in medium saucepan. Add rice. Cover tightly and cook over low heat until all liquid is absorbed, about 50 minutes. About 15 minutes before rice is cooked, combine tarragon, salt and pepper. Sprinkle over chicken; rub seasoning onto top and bottom surfaces. Cook chicken in margarine in 12-inch non-stick skillet over medium heat until cooked through, about 7 minutes per side. Stir red pepper and almonds into rice. To serve, arrange chicken over rice. Sprinkle green onions on top.

Makes 6 servings

Per Serving: *300 calories, 31 g protein, 6 g fat, 26 g carbohydrate, 400 mg sodium*

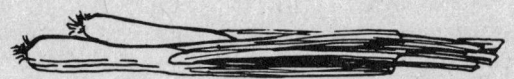

WESTERN BEANS AND RICE

   1 cup chopped onion
   1 cup sliced celery
   1 tablespoon vegetable oil
   3 cups drained cooked or canned pinto beans
   1 can (8 ounces) tomato sauce
   ½ cup water
   ½ teaspoon salt
   ⅛ to ¼ teaspoon hot pepper sauce
   3 cups cooked brown rice*

Cook onion and celery in oil in large skillet until tender. Stir in beans, tomato sauce, water, salt, and hot pepper sauce; heat through. Serve over rice.
Makes 6 servings

*Prepared without butter or salt.

Per Serving: 250 calories, 10 g protein, 3 g fat, 45 g carbohydrate, 420 mg sodium

CHICKEN MARENGO

   ½ teaspoon garlic powder
   ½ teaspoon salt
   ½ teaspoon dried marjoram, crushed
   ½ teaspoon dried thyme, crushed
   ½ teaspoon freshly ground pepper
   6 chicken breast halves, boned and skinned
   1 can (14½ or 16 ounces) whole tomatoes
   ½ cup dry white wine
   1 medium onion, cut into wedges
   1 cup UNCLE BEN'S® CONVERTED® Brand Rice
   ¼ cup pimiento-stuffed green olives, sliced

Combine garlic powder, salt, marjoram, thyme and pepper. Sprinkle over both sides of chicken. Drain and coarsely chop tomatoes, reserving liquid. If necessary, add enough water to liquid to equal 1½ cups. Combine tomato liquid and wine in

10-inch skillet. Bring to a boil. Stir in onion and rice. Arrange chicken over rice, pressing down into rice. Arrange tomatoes over chicken. Cover tightly and simmer 20 minutes. Remove from heat. Let stand covered until all liquid is absorbed, about 5 minutes. Sprinkle with olives.

Makes 6 servings

Per Serving: 285 calories, 30 g protein, 2 g fat, 31 g carbohydrate, 394 mg sodium

CHILI-CHEESE RICE QUICHE

2 large eggs, beaten
1 cup skim milk
¼ teaspoon garlic salt
Freshly ground pepper, to taste
1 cup cooked and cooled UNCLE BEN'S® CONVERTED® Brand Rice*
¾ cup (3 ounces) shredded low-moisture, part-skim mozzarella cheese
¼ cup chopped onion
2 tablespoons chopped pimiento
1 to 2 tablespoons diced jalapeño peppers
1 tablespoon grated Parmesan cheese

Combine eggs, milk, garlic salt and pepper in mixing bowl; mix well. Stir in rice, mozzarella cheese, onion, pimiento and jalapeño peppers. Pour into 8-inch glass pie plate coated with vegetable oil cooking spray. Bake at 350°F. for 30 to 35 minutes or until knife inserted near center comes out clean. Sprinkle with Parmesan cheese. Let stand 10 minutes.

Makes 2 servings

*Prepared without butter or salt.

Per Serving: 345 calories, 25 g protein, 14 g fat, 28 g carbohydrate, 602 mg sodium when prepared with 1 tablespoon jalapeño peppers

QUICK CHICKEN-SHRIMP GUMBO

- ½ cup diced green pepper
- ⅓ cup chopped onion
- 2 tablespoons margarine
- ¼ cup flour
- 1 can (28 ounces) whole tomatoes
- 2 cups diced cooked chicken
- 1 teaspoon salt
- 1 teaspoon dried thyme
- ¼ teaspoon hot pepper sauce
- ½ pound medium shrimp, peeled and deveined
- 2 tablespoons chopped parsley
- 3½ cups hot cooked UNCLE BEN'S® CONVERTED® Brand Rice*

Cook green pepper and onion in margarine in large saucepan until tender but not brown. Stir in flour. Add tomatoes, chicken, salt, thyme and hot pepper sauce. Break up tomatoes with spoon. Cover and simmer 20 minutes. Add shrimp and continue cooking 5 minutes. Stir parsley into hot cooked rice. To serve, spoon gumbo into individual serving bowls; top with rice.

Makes 6 servings

*Prepared without butter or salt.

Per Serving: *290 calories, 25 g protein, 7 g fat, 31 g carbohydrate, 664 mg sodium*

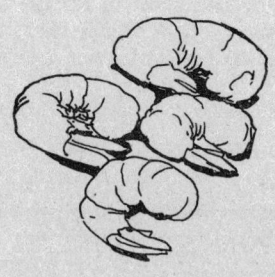

MONTEREY FISH AND BROWN RICE

2⅔ cups water
1 teaspoon salt (optional)
1 cup UNCLE BEN'S® Select Brown Rice
½ cup coarsely chopped celery
3 garlic cloves, minced
2 teaspoons vegetable oil
1 cup dry white wine
¼ cup tomato paste
1 teaspoon dried thyme, crushed
1½ pounds fresh cod fillets, cut into serving-size pieces*
½ cup very thinly sliced mushrooms
1 small tomato, chopped
2 tablespoons chopped green onions with tops
¼ cup sliced ripe olives

Bring water and, if desired, salt to a boil in medium saucepan. Stir in rice and celery. Cover tightly and cook over low heat until all water is absorbed, about 50 minutes. About 15 minutes before serving, cook garlic in oil in large non-stick skillet until tender. Add wine, tomato paste and thyme; stir to mix well. Add fish. Cook over medium-low heat, 10 to 12 minutes, or until fish flakes when tested with a fork. Stir mushrooms, tomato and onion into rice. Arrange fish over rice; pour sauce over. Sprinkle with olives.

Makes 6 servings

*1½ pounds frozen cod fillets, thawed, may be substituted.

Per Serving: *330 calories, 29 g protein, 10 g fat, 29 g carbohydrate, 553 mg sodium when prepared with salt*

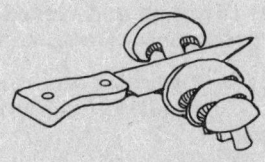

SHRIMP FRIED RICE

   1 tablespoon vegetable oil
   2 eggs, slightly beaten
   ¼ teaspoon pepper
3½ cups cooked and cooled UNCLE BEN'S®
       CONVERTED® Brand Rice*
   2 cups small cooked shrimp
   2 tablespoons soy sauce
   ½ cup chopped green onions with tops

Heat oil in 10-inch non-stick skillet over medium heat. Add eggs and pepper. Cook 5 minutes, stirring frequently, until eggs are set. Add cooked rice, shrimp and soy sauce. Cook, stirring frequently, 5 minutes longer. Stir in green onions.
Makes 4 servings

*Prepared without butter or salt.

Per Serving: 285 calories, 22 g protein, 7 g fat, 32 g carbohydrate, 626 mg sodium

TURKEY ORIENTAL SOUP

3½ cups turkey or chicken broth
3½ cups water
   ⅔ cup uncooked rice
   4 cups (1¼ pounds) coarsely chopped cooked
       turkey
   1 cup diagonally sliced celery
   2 medium carrots, cut into matchstick strips
   2 tablespoons reduced sodium soy sauce
   2 tablespoons dry sherry
1½ teaspoons cornstarch
   1 can (14 ounces) fancy mixed Chinese
       vegetables, drained and rinsed
   ½ cup sliced green onions with tops

Combine turkey broth, water and rice in 4-quart saucepan. Bring to a boil. Reduce heat and simmer

10 minutes. Add turkey, celery and carrots. Simmer 5 minutes. Combine soy sauce, sherry and cornstarch. Add to saucepan with mixed vegetables and onions. Simmer, stirring occasionally, until soup is clear and slightly thickened.

Makes 10 servings

Per Serving: *170 calories, 19 g protein, 4 g fat, 13 g carbohydrate, 395 mg sodium*

MEXICAN CHICKEN WITH JALAPEÑO RICE

- 1 teaspoon each: chili powder, ground cumin
- 2 large chicken breast halves, boned and skinned (about ¾ pound)
- 1¼ cups chicken broth
- ½ cup UNCLE BEN'S® CONVERTED® Brand Rice
- ⅓ cup coarsely chopped onion
- ¼ cup canned diced green chilies
- 1 small tomato, seeded and diced
- 2 tablespoons plain low-fat yogurt
- 1 tablespoon chopped cilantro

Combine chili powder and cumin, reserving ½ teaspoon. Rub remaining seasoning mixture onto chicken breast halves; set aside. Bring chicken broth to a boil in 10-inch skillet. Stir in rice, onion, chilies and reserved seasonings. Arrange chicken breasts on top. Cover tightly and simmer 20 minutes. Remove from heat. Stir in tomato. Let stand covered until all liquid is absorbed, about 5 minutes. Spoon yogurt over chicken. Sprinkle with cilantro.

Makes 2 servings

Per Serving: *350 calories, 35 g protein, 2 g fat, 47 g carbohydrate, 561 mg sodium*

SCALLOP SAUTE WITH CURRIED RICE

1⅓ cups chicken broth
½ cup UNCLE BEN'S® CONVERTED® Brand Rice
1 teaspoon curry powder
¾ teaspoon sugar
¼ teaspoon turmeric
½ pound bay scallops*
1 large garlic clove, minced
¼ teaspoon red pepper flakes
2 teaspoons margarine
½ cup seeded, diced tomato
1 tablespoon toasted slivered almonds
1 tablespoon minced parsley

Bring chicken broth to a boil in small saucepan. Stir in rice, curry powder, sugar and turmeric. Cover tightly and simmer 20 minutes. Remove from heat. Let stand covered while preparing scallops. Saute scallops, garlic and red pepper flakes in margarine in small non-stick skillet 2 to 3 minutes or until cooked through. Remove from heat. Stir tomato and almonds into rice. Spoon scallops over rice. Sprinkle with parsley.

Makes 2 servings

*Sea scallops, cut in half, may be substituted.

Per Serving: *365 calories, 25 g protein, 7 g fat, 50 g carbohydrate, 823 mg sodium*

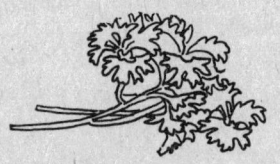

CHINATOWN CHICKEN AND ZUCCHINI

- 1 cup UNCLE BEN'S® Select Brown Rice
- 2 whole chicken breasts, boned and skinned
- 2 teaspoons vegetable oil
- 1 garlic clove, minced
- 3 medium zucchini, cut into ¼-inch slices
- 1 can (8 ounces) water chestnuts, drained and sliced
- 2 to 3 tablespoons soy sauce
- ½ cup water
- 1 tablespoon cornstarch
- ⅓ cup sliced green onions with tops

Prepare rice according to package directions omitting butter and salt. Cut chicken breasts into 1½×½×½-inch strips. About 20 minutes before rice is cooked, heat oil in large non-stick skillet. Add chicken and garlic. Cook and stir over medium-high heat 2 to 3 minutes. Add zucchini, water chestnuts and soy sauce. Cover and cook until zucchini is crisp-tender, 2 to 3 minutes. Combine water and cornstarch; add to skillet. Cook, stirring frequently, until mixture is thickened and clear, about 2 minutes. Stir green onions into hot cooked rice. Serve chicken mixture over rice.

Makes 6 servings

Per Serving: *255 calories, 22 g protein, 3 g fat, 33 g carbohydrate, 400 mg sodium when prepared with 2 tablespoons soy sauce*

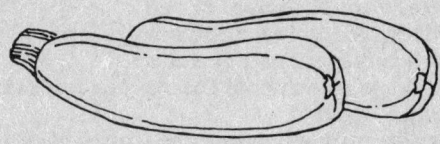

SHRIMP AND RICE VERACRUZ

  1 can (14½ or 16 ounces) whole tomatoes
  1 cup coarsely chopped onion
  3 large garlic cloves, minced
  1 cup UNCLE BEN'S® CONVERTED® Brand Rice
  2 bay leaves
  ½ cup small pimiento-stuffed green olives
  1 teaspoon salt (optional)
  1 pound cooked and cleaned medium shrimp
  1 large green pepper, cut into 2×¼-inch strips
  1 tablespoon capers

Drain and chop tomatoes, reserving liquid. Add enough water to liquid to equal 2½ cups. Combine tomato liquid, tomatoes, onion and garlic in large skillet. Bring to a boil. Stir in rice, bay leaves, olives and, if desired, salt. Cover tightly and simmer 20 minutes. Stir in shrimp, green pepper and capers. Remove from heat. Let stand covered until all liquid is absorbed, about 5 minutes. Remove bay leaves.

Makes 6 servings

Per Serving: *240 calories, 22 g protein, 2 g fat, 33 g carbohydrate, 650 mg sodium when prepared with salt*

SAN FRANCISCO PORK FRIED RICE

  1 cup UNCLE BEN'S® Select Brown Rice
  2 teaspoons vegetable oil
  ¾ pound boneless pork, cut into thin strips
  1 garlic clove, minced
  ½ pound mushrooms, sliced
  ½ cup sliced green onions with tops
  2 to 3 tablespoons soy sauce
  1 package (6 ounces) frozen pea pods, thawed and drained
  1 can (8 ounces) water chestnuts, drained and sliced

Prepare rice according to package directions omitting butter and salt; cover and chill. Heat oil in large non-stick skillet. Add pork and garlic. Cook and stir over medium-high heat until pork is well browned. Add mushrooms. Cook and stir about 2 minutes. Add rice, green onions and soy sauce. Cook and stir until heated through. Stir in pea pods and water chestnuts.

Makes 6 servings

Per Serving: 315 calories, 13 g protein, 14 g fat, 33 g carbohydrate, 386 mg sodium when prepared with 2 tablespoons soy sauce

PICANTE CHICKEN 'N RICE

6 chicken breast halves, boned and skinned
Salt, to taste (optional)
¾ cup coarsely chopped onion
3 large garlic cloves, minced
2 teaspoons vegetable oil
1¼ cups chicken broth
1 cup medium red salsa or picante sauce
1 cup UNCLE BEN'S® CONVERTED® Brand Rice
1 medium tomato, coarsely chopped
¼ cup (1 ounce) shredded cheddar or Monterey Jack cheese
¼ cup sliced ripe olives

Sprinkle chicken breasts with salt; set aside. Cook onion and garlic in oil in 10-inch non-stick skillet 2 minutes. Add chicken broth and salsa. Bring to a boil. Stir in rice. Arrange chicken breasts over rice. Cover tightly and simmer 20 minutes. Remove from heat. Let stand covered until all liquid is absorbed, about 5 minutes. Garnish with tomato, cheese and olives.

Makes 6 servings

Per Serving: 315 calories, 32 g protein, 5 g fat, 32 g carbohydrate, 517 mg sodium when prepared without salt

FISH KABOBS & ZUCCHINI BROWN RICE

- ¼ cup finely chopped onion
- 2 tablespoons finely chopped celery
- 1 garlic clove, minced
- 1 tablespoon margarine
- 2⅔ cups water
- 1 cup UNCLE BEN'S® Select Brown Rice
- 1 teaspoon salt (optional)
- 1 cup chili sauce
- 2 tablespoons dry red wine
- 1 tablespoon vegetable oil
- ¼ to ½ teaspoon red pepper flakes
- 1½ pounds cod fillets, fresh or frozen, cut into 1½-inch cubes
- 1 jar (2 ounces) chopped pimiento, drained
- 1 medium zucchini, chopped
- ½ teaspoon dried basil, crushed
- Lime wedges

Saute onion, celery and garlic in margarine in large saucepan until tender. Add water; bring to a boil. Add rice and, if desired, salt. Cover tightly and cook over low heat until all water is absorbed, about 50 minutes. Combine chili sauce, wine, oil and red pepper flakes; mix well. Pour over fish cubes in shallow baking dish. Marinate 20 minutes, turning occasionally. Thread fish cubes on 6 wooden or metal skewers. Brush with marinade. Cook 4 to 6 inches from heat source, 7 to 9 minutes, or until fish flakes when tested with a fork. Turn once and baste during cooking. Stir pimiento, zucchini and basil into rice. To serve, spoon rice onto serving platter. Place lime wedge on the end of each skewer. Arrange kabobs over rice.

Makes 6 servings

Per Serving: 300 calories, 24 g protein, 5 g fat, 37 g carbohydrate, 1064 mg sodium when prepared with salt

POLYNESIAN CHICKEN AND RICE

1½ pounds boned and skinned chicken breasts, cut into 1½-inch pieces
  Pepper, to taste
2 tablespoons cornstarch, divided
1 can (16 ounces) sliced peaches, packed in juice
1 medium onion, thinly sliced
1 tablespoon vegetable oil
1 can (8 ounces) no-salt-added tomato sauce
2 tablespoons reduced sodium soy sauce
1 medium green pepper, coarsely chopped
3 cups hot cooked rice*

Sprinkle chicken with pepper and 1 tablespoon of the cornstarch. Drain peaches, reserving juice. Cook chicken and onion in oil in large non-stick skillet until chicken is lightly browned. Combine reserved peach juice, tomato sauce, soy sauce and remaining 1 tablespoon cornstarch; add to skillet. Cook, stirring constantly, until thickened and bubbly. Add green pepper and peaches. Simmer 5 minutes or until pepper is crisp-tender. Serve over rice.

Makes 6 servings

*Prepared without butter or salt.

Per Serving: *300 calories, 29 g protein, 4 g fat, 37 g carbohydrate, 297 mg sodium*

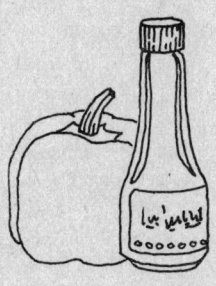

GINGERED SHRIMP AND SPRING RICE

1⅓ cups water
½ cup UNCLE BEN'S® CONVERTED® Brand Rice
1 to 2 tablespoons soy sauce
¼ pound fresh asparagus, cut into 1-inch pieces*
¼ cup diced red or green pepper
2 teaspoons vegetable oil
½ pound medium shrimp, peeled and deveined, with tails left on
2 garlic cloves, minced
1½ teaspoons finely grated fresh ginger
Red pepper flakes, to taste
¼ cup dry white wine

Bring water to a boil in small saucepan. Stir in rice and soy sauce. Cover tightly and simmer 20 minutes. Remove from heat. Stir in asparagus and diced red pepper. Let stand covered while preparing shrimp. Heat oil in medium non-stick skillet. Add shrimp, garlic, ginger and red pepper flakes. Cook, stirring constantly, 2 minutes. Add wine. Continue cooking and stirring over medium heat until shrimp are cooked through. Serve over rice.

Makes 2 servings

*¾ cup frozen cut asparagus, thawed, may be substituted.

Per Serving: *365 calories, 26 g protein, 6 g fat, 45 g carbohydrate, 682 mg sodium when prepared with 1 tablespoon soy sauce*

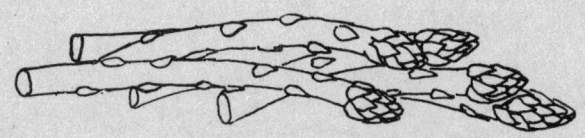

TRI-COLORED SALMON BAKE

2½ cups water
1 cup UNCLE BEN'S® CONVERTED® Brand Rice
1½ teaspoons salt
2 tablespoons margarine
2 tablespoons flour
2 cups chicken broth
2 teaspoons lemon juice
¼ teaspoon pepper
2 tablespoons minced onion
1 teaspoon dried dill weed
1 can (15½ ounces) salmon, drained and flaked
1 package (10 ounces) frozen chopped spinach, thawed and well drained
Green onions (optional)
Pimiento (optional)

Bring water to a boil in medium saucepan. Stir in rice and 1 teaspoon of the salt. Cover tightly and simmer 20 minutes. While rice is cooking, melt margarine in medium saucepan. Stir in flour. Cook and stir 2 minutes. Gradually stir in chicken broth. Bring to a boil, stirring constantly. Add lemon juice, pepper and the remaining ½ teaspoon salt. Reduce heat. Cook, stirring occasionally, 5 minutes. Remove rice from heat. Let stand covered until all water is absorbed, about 5 minutes. Stir ½ cup sauce, onion and dill weed into salmon. Stir ¼ cup sauce into spinach. Stir remaining sauce into rice. Spoon about 2 cups rice into 1½-quart souffle dish or casserole. Spread spinach evenly over rice. Spoon salmon evenly over spinach. Spread remaining rice evenly over salmon. Cover and bake at 325°F. for 20 minutes. Garnish with green onions and pimiento, if desired.

Makes 6 servings

Per Serving: *300 calories, 19 g protein, 12 g fat, 29 g carbohydrate, 1146 mg sodium when prepared without garnishes*

ORIENTAL VEGETABLE AND LAMB SKILLET

1 tablespoon vegetable oil
1 pound lamb cubes, trimmed of visible fat
2 garlic cloves, minced
1 can (10¾ ounces) condensed chicken broth
1 cup UNCLE BEN'S® Select Brown Rice
¼ teaspoon red pepper flakes
1 cup broccoli flowerets
1 cup cauliflower flowerets
1 small red pepper, cut into thin strips
1 teaspoon finely shredded fresh ginger
1 teaspoon sesame oil

Heat vegetable oil in 10-inch non-stick skillet. Add lamb and garlic; brown evenly. Drain excess fat. Add enough water to chicken broth to equal 2⅔ cups. Bring to a boil in skillet. Stir in rice and red pepper flakes. Cover tightly and cook over low heat 40 minutes. Add broccoli and cauliflower. Cover and continue cooking until all liquid is absorbed and vegetables are tender, about 10 minutes. Stir in red pepper strips, ginger and sesame oil. *Makes 6 servings*

Per Serving: 300 calories, 26 g protein, 9 g fat, 27 g carbohydrate, 361 mg sodium

TUNA CREOLE SKILLET

1 can (14½ or 16 ounces) stewed tomatoes
½ cup chopped green pepper
2 teaspoons margarine
1 cup UNCLE BEN'S® CONVERTED® Brand Rice
1 tablespoon instant minced onion
1 teaspoon salt (optional)
1 can (6½ or 7 ounces) tuna, packed in water, drained and flaked

Drain tomatoes, reserving liquid. Add enough water to liquid to equal 2½ cups; set aside. Cook green pepper in margarine in large non-stick skillet 2 to 3 minutes. Add rice, onion, salt, if desired, tomato liquid and reserved tomatoes to skillet. Bring to a boil. Reduce heat. Cover tightly and simmer 20 minutes. Remove from heat and stir in tuna. Let stand covered until all liquid is absorbed, about 5 minutes.

Makes 4 servings

Per Serving: *290 calories, 18 g protein, 3 g fat, 47 g carbohydrate, 884 mg sodium when prepared with salt*

BEEF AND RICE PROVENCAL

- 1 pound beef top round or sirloin, trimmed of visible fat and cut into strips
- 1 medium onion, thinly sliced
- 2 garlic cloves, minced
- 1 tablespoon vegetable oil
- 1 can (14½ or 16 ounces) whole tomatoes
- 1 cup UNCLE BEN'S® CONVERTED® Brand Rice
- ¼ pound mushrooms, quartered
- 2 medium carrots, diagonally sliced ¼-inch thick
- 2 teaspoons instant beef bouillon granules
- 1 teaspoon salt (optional)
- ½ teaspoon dried sage

Brown beef with onion and garlic in oil in large non-stick skillet over medium heat. Drain and coarsely chop tomatoes, reserving liquid. Add enough water to liquid to equal 2¼ cups. Add liquid, rice, tomatoes, mushrooms, carrots, bouillon, salt, if desired, and sage to skillet. Bring to a boil. Reduce heat. Cover tightly and simmer until most of the liquid is absorbed and meat is tender, 25 to 30 minutes.

Makes 6 servings

Per Serving: *390 calories, 16 g protein, 21 g fat, 34 g carbohydrate, 527 mg sodium when prepared with salt*

EGGS RANCHERO BROWN RICE CASSEROLE

1 can (14½ or 16 ounces) whole tomatoes
1 cup UNCLE BEN'S® Select Brown Rice
1 teaspoon chili powder
1 teaspoon salt (optional)
1 can (4 ounces) chopped green chilies, drained
3 green onions with tops, sliced
5 eggs
Pepper, as desired
½ cup (2 ounces) shredded low-moisture, part-skim mozzarella cheese

Coarsely chop and drain tomatoes, reserving liquid. Add enough water to liquid to equal 2⅔ cups. Bring to a boil in medium saucepan. Add rice, chili powder and, if desired, salt. Cover tightly and cook over low heat until all liquid is absorbed, about 50 minutes. Stir in chilies, green onions and tomatoes. Spoon into 11×7×2-inch baking dish. Make five indentations in rice mixture with back of spoon.* Break an egg into each indentation. Sprinkle eggs with pepper. Bake uncovered at 325°F. for 10 minutes. Sprinkle with cheese. Continue baking until eggs are as done as desired.

Makes 5 servings

*At this point, casserole may be covered tightly with foil and refrigerated up to 24 hours. When ready to serve, uncover and continue assembling casserole as above. Bake uncovered at 350°F. for 25 minutes. Sprinkle with cheese. Continue baking until eggs are as done as desired.

Per Serving: 280 calories, 13 g protein, 9 g fat, 36 g carbohydrate, 682 mg sodium when rice is prepared with salt

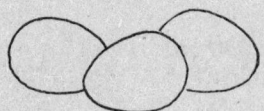

CREOLE FISH 'N RICE SKILLET

   2 flounder or sole fillets (½ pound)
   ¼ teaspoon salt (optional)
   1 can (8¼ ounces) whole tomatoes
   ½ cup UNCLE BEN'S® CONVERTED® Brand Rice
   ½ cup coarsely chopped onion
   2 garlic cloves, minced
   1 tablespoon lemon juice
   1¼ teaspoons dried basil, crushed
   ½ teaspoon dried oregano, crushed
   ⅛ teaspoon hot pepper sauce
      Freshly ground pepper, to taste
   1 small carrot, shredded
   ½ green pepper, cut into matchstick strips

Sprinkle fish fillets with salt, if desired. Roll up, securing with wooden picks; set aside. Drain and coarsely chop tomatoes, reserving liquid. Add enough water to liquid to equal 1⅓ cups. Bring to a boil in 10-inch skillet. Stir in tomatoes, rice, onion, garlic, lemon juice, basil, oregano, hot pepper sauce and pepper. Arrange fish fillets on top. Cover tightly and simmer 20 minutes. Remove from heat. Sprinkle carrot and green pepper over fish. Let stand covered until all liquid is absorbed and fish flakes when tested with a fork, about 5 minutes.

Makes 2 servings

Per Serving: *330 calories, 25 g protein, 2 g fat, 52 g carbohydrate, 265 mg sodium when prepared without salt*

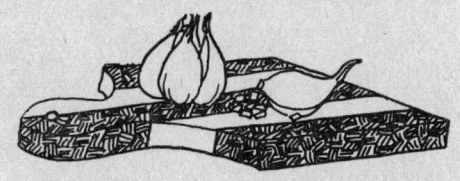

Main Dishes

SOLE ROLL-UPS

12 small sole or other thin fish fillets (1½ pounds)
1½ teaspoons salt
⅛ teaspoon white pepper
1½ cups shredded carrot
2 tablespoons chopped green onions with tops
1½ tablespoons margarine, melted
2 teaspoons lemon juice
2½ cups water
1 cup UNCLE BEN'S® CONVERTED® Brand Rice
2 tablespoons finely chopped parsley
Paprika

Thaw fish, if frozen. Sprinkle ¾ teaspoon of the salt and the white pepper evenly over fillets; set aside. Cook carrot and green onion in ½ tablespoon of the margarine in skillet over low heat until carrots are tender, about 10 minutes. Spread an equal amount of carrot mixture on each fillet and roll up. Arrange seam side down in 13×9×2-inch baking dish. Combine remaining 1 tablespoon margarine with lemon juice; drizzle over fish rolls. Bake uncovered at 350°F. until fish flakes when tested with a fork, 25 to 30 minutes. Meanwhile, bring water to a boil in medium saucepan. Stir in rice and remaining ¾ teaspoon salt. Cover tightly and simmer 20 minutes. Remove from heat. Let stand covered until all water is absorbed, about 5 minutes. Stir in parsley. Arrange fish and rice on platter. Sprinkle with paprika.

Makes 6 servings

Per Serving: 250 calories, 22 g protein, 4 g fat, 30 g carbohydrate, 678 mg sodium

Side Dishes

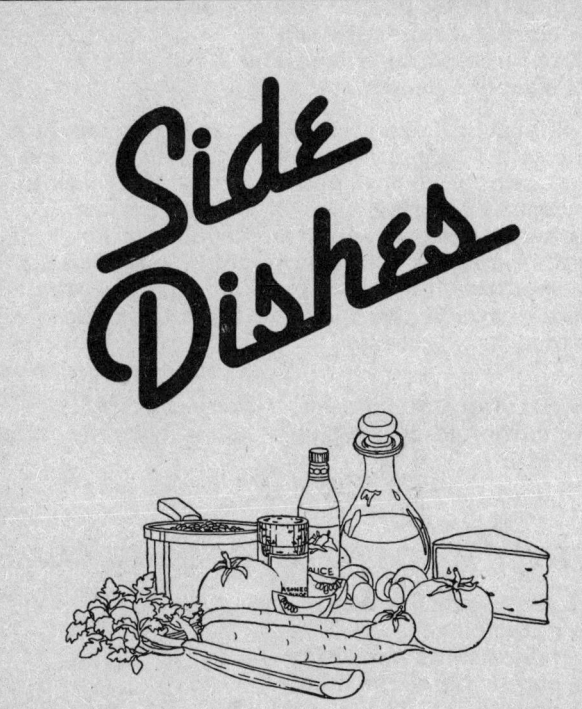

LEMONY ZUCCHINI BROWN RICE

- 1 small zucchini, cut into 1×⅛×⅛-inch strips
- 1 to 2 garlic cloves, minced
- 2 teaspoons margarine
- 1 cup fresh spinach leaves, cut into 1×¼-inch strips
- 2⅔ cups water
- 1 cup UNCLE BEN'S® Select Brown Rice
- 1 teaspoon salt (optional)
- 2 to 3 teaspoons lemon juice
- ⅛ teaspoon pepper

Cook zucchini and garlic in margarine in medium saucepan 1 to 2 minutes. Add spinach. Cook and stir 1 minute; remove and set aside. Add water to saucepan and bring to a boil. Stir in rice and, if desired, salt. Cover tightly and cook over low heat until all water is absorbed, about 50 minutes. Stir reserved zucchini and spinach, lemon juice and pepper into rice. Remove from heat. Let stand covered 2 to 3 minutes.

Makes 6 servings

Per Serving: 130 calories, 3 g protein, 2 g fat, 25 g carbohydrate, 380 mg sodium when prepared with salt

WHITE RISOTTO WITH MUSHROOMS

- ½ pound mushrooms, sliced
- 1 garlic clove
- 1½ tablespoons margarine
- 1 cup thinly sliced onion
- 1 cup UNCLE BEN'S® CONVERTED® Brand Rice
- 2¼ cups chicken broth
- ¼ cup dry white wine
- 1 teaspoon salt
- ¼ teaspoon white pepper
- ¼ cup freshly grated Parmesan cheese
- 2 tablespoons chopped parsley

Cook mushrooms and garlic in 1 tablespoon of the margarine in 10-inch non-stick skillet until mushrooms are tender but not brown. Remove mushrooms with slotted spoon and reserve; discard garlic. Add remaining ½ tablespoon margarine to skillet. Add onion and rice. Cook over medium-high heat, stirring constantly, 3 to 4 minutes or until rice is translucent. Add chicken broth, wine, salt, pepper and reserved mushrooms. Bring to a boil. Reduce heat. Cover tightly and simmer 20 minutes. Remove from heat. Stir in cheese and parsley. Let stand covered until all liquid is absorbed, about 5 minutes.

Makes 8 servings

Per Serving: 140 calories, 5 g protein, 3 g fat, 23 g carbohydrate, 551 mg sodium

HARVEST RICE

1 cup sliced carrots
3 tablespoons vegetable oil
2 cups chopped unpeeled apples
1 cup sliced green onions with tops
3 cups cooked brown rice*
½ cup raisins
½ teaspoon salt
1 tablespoon sesame seeds

Cook carrots in oil in large skillet over medium heat about 5 minutes. Add apples and onions. Cook and stir 5 minutes. Stir in rice, raisins and salt. Continue cooking and stirring until rice is heated through. Add sesame seeds; toss lightly.

Makes 8 servings

*Prepared without butter or salt.

Per Serving: 190 calories, 2 g protein, 6 g fat, 30 g carbohydrate, 200 mg sodium

GAZPACHO-STYLE RICE

2½ cups water
1 tablespoon chicken bouillon granules
1 cup UNCLE BEN'S® CONVERTED® Brand Rice
2 green onions with tops, sliced
1 garlic clove, minced
1½ tablespoons olive oil
1 tablespoon red wine vinegar
½ teaspoon salt
Dash pepper
1 medium tomato, chopped
1 medium green pepper, chopped
1 small cucumber, chopped

Combine water and bouillon granules in medium saucepan; bring to a boil. Stir in rice. Cover tightly and simmer 20 minutes. Meanwhile, combine green onions, garlic, oil, vinegar, salt and pepper; mix well. Stir into hot cooked rice. Serve bowls of tomato, green pepper and cucumber separately. Sprinkle vegetables over rice as desired.
Makes 6 servings

Per Serving: 165 calories, 3 g protein, 4 g fat, 29 g carbohydrate, 200 mg sodium

MIDDLE EASTERN PILAF

½ cup chopped onion
1 tablespoon margarine
1 tablespoon olive oil
1 cup UNCLE BEN'S® CONVERTED® Brand Rice
⅓ cup slivered almonds
2½ cups chicken broth
1 teaspoon salt (optional)
¼ teaspoon pepper
¼ cup golden raisins
2 tablespoons chopped parsley
1½ teaspoons chopped fresh mint leaves OR ½ teaspoon dried mint leaves

Cook onion in margarine and oil in medium saucepan until tender, about 5 minutes. Add rice and almonds. Cook over low heat, stirring constantly, until rice is golden. Add chicken broth, salt, if desired, and pepper. Bring to a boil. Reduce heat. Cover tightly and simmer 20 minutes. Remove from heat and stir in remaining ingredients. Let stand covered until all liquid is absorbed, about 5 minutes.

Makes 8 servings

Per Serving: *170 calories, 4 g protein, 6 g fat, 25 g carbohydrate, 513 mg sodium when prepared with salt*

VEGETABLE BROWN RICE CURRY

- 1 medium onion, cut into ¼-inch wedges
- 1 garlic clove, minced
- 2 teaspoons margarine
- 1 can (13¾ or 14½ ounces) chicken broth
- 1 cup UNCLE BEN'S® Select Brown Rice
- 1 tablespoon honey
- 1 teaspoon curry powder
- ¼ pound carrots, cut into 1×¼×¼-inch strips
- ½ cup raisins
- ⅓ cup dry roasted peanuts

Cook onion and garlic in margarine in 10-inch nonstick skillet over medium heat until onion is tender but not brown. Add enough water to chicken broth to equal 2⅔ cups. Add to skillet and bring to a boil. Add rice, honey and curry powder. Cover tightly and cook over low heat 45 minutes. Add carrots and raisins. Cover and continue cooking until all liquid is absorbed, about 5 minutes. Stir in peanuts.

Makes 8 servings

Per Serving: *190 calories, 4 g protein, 5 g fat, 32 g carbohydrate, 250 mg sodium*

BROWN RICE AND SPROUTS ORIENTAL

  3 tablespoons white vinegar
  2 tablespoons soy sauce
  1 cup UNCLE BEN'S® Select Brown Rice
2½ teaspoons sugar
  2 teaspoons margarine
  3 medium carrots, cut diagonally into
     ⅛-inch slices
  1 pound fresh bean sprouts, rinsed and drained*
  4 green onions with tops, cut into 1-inch pieces

Combine vinegar and soy sauce. Add enough water to equal 2⅔ cups. Bring to a boil in 10-inch skillet. Stir in rice, sugar and margarine. Cover tightly and cook over low heat 35 minutes. Top with carrots. Cover and continue cooking until all liquid is absorbed, about 15 minutes. Stir in bean sprouts and green onions; heat through.

Makes 6 servings

*1 can (16 ounces) bean sprouts, drained and rinsed, may be substituted.

Per Serving: *185 calories, 6 g protein, 2 g fat, 35 g carbohydrate, 382 mg sodium*

GARDEN VEGETABLE SAUTE WITH BROWN RICE

  ½ pound green beans, cut into 1-inch pieces
  1 cup small cauliflower flowerets
  2 garlic cloves, minced
  1 tablespoon margarine
2⅔ cups water
  1 cup UNCLE BEN'S® Select Brown Rice
  1 teaspoon salt (optional)
  ½ teaspoon paprika
  ⅛ teaspoon cayenne pepper
  ¼ cup plain low-fat yogurt, at room temperature

Cook green beans, cauliflower and garlic in margarine in 10-inch non-stick skillet over medium heat until vegetables are crisp-tender, 7 to 10 minutes. Remove vegetables and set aside. Add water to skillet and bring to a boil. Stir in rice, salt, if desired, paprika and cayenne pepper. Cover tightly and cook over low heat 45 minutes. Add vegetables. Cover and continue cooking over low heat until all water is absorbed, about 5 minutes. Remove from heat; stir in yogurt.

Makes 6 servings

Per Serving: 150 calories, 4 g protein, 2 g fat, 28 g carbohydrate, 391 mg sodium when prepared with salt

MONTEREY RISOTTO

1 tablespoon margarine
1 cup sliced mushrooms
¼ cup chopped onion
1 cup UNCLE BEN'S® CONVERTED® Brand Rice
2 cups chicken broth
½ cup dry white wine
1 teaspoon salt (optional)
½ cup (2 ounces) shredded Monterey Jack cheese

Melt margarine in medium saucepan. Add mushrooms and onion. Cook, stirring occasionally, until golden. Add rice, chicken broth, wine and, if desired, salt; stir. Bring to a boil. Reduce heat. Cover tightly and simmer 20 minutes. Remove from heat. Let stand covered until all liquid is absorbed, about 5 minutes. Stir in cheese.

Makes 6 servings

Per Serving: 185 calories, 6 g protein, 5 g fat, 28 g carbohydrate, 675 mg sodium when prepared with salt

COUNTRY-STYLE SUMMER VEGETABLE RICE

- 1 cup UNCLE BEN'S® CONVERTED® Brand Rice
- 2 garlic cloves, minced
- 1 tablespoon margarine
- 2½ cups water
- 1¼ teaspoons dried basil, crushed
- 1¼ teaspoons salt
- 1 small zucchini, cut into 1×⅛×⅛-inch strips
- 1 small yellow squash, cut into 1×⅛×⅛-inch strips
- 1 small tomato, cut into ½-inch pieces

Cook rice and garlic in margarine in medium saucepan over low heat until rice is lightly browned, 5 to 7 minutes. Add water, basil and salt. Bring to a boil. Reduce heat. Cover tightly and simmer 20 minutes. Stir in zucchini, yellow squash and tomato. Remove from heat. Let stand covered until all water is absorbed, about 5 minutes.

Makes 6 servings

Per Serving: 145 calories, 3 g protein, 2 g fat, 28 g carbohydrate, 471 mg sodium

CURRIED ORANGE 'N PEAR RICE

- 1½ cups orange juice
- 1 cup water
- 1 cup UNCLE BEN'S® CONVERTED® Brand Rice
- 2 teaspoons margarine
- 1¼ teaspoons curry powder
- ½ teaspoon salt
- 2 medium pears, coarsely chopped
- ¼ cup coarsely chopped pecans
- 2 tablespoons chutney, chopped

Bring orange juice and water to a boil in medium saucepan. Stir in rice, margarine, curry powder and salt. Cover tightly and simmer 20 minutes. Remove from heat. Stir in pears, nuts and chutney. Let stand covered until all liquid is absorbed, about 5 minutes.

Makes 8 servings

Per Serving: *180 calories, 3 g protein, 4 g fat, 33 g carbohydrate, 156 mg sodium*

ORIENTAL RICE PILAF

2½ cups chicken broth
1 cup UNCLE BEN'S® CONVERTED® Brand Rice
2 to 3 tablespoons soy sauce
½ teaspoon salt (optional)
⅛ to ¼ teaspoon ground ginger
3 cups coarsely shredded cabbage
½ cup sliced green onions with tops
½ cup thinly sliced carrots

Combine chicken broth, rice, soy sauce, salt, if desired, and ginger in 10-inch skillet. Bring to a boil. Reduce heat. Cover tightly and simmer 20 minutes. Remove from heat and stir in remaining ingredients. Let stand covered until all liquid is absorbed, about 5 minutes.

Makes 8 servings

Per Serving: *115 calories, 4 g protein, less than 1 g fat, 24 g carbohydrate, 631 mg sodium when prepared with salt and 2 tablespoons soy sauce*

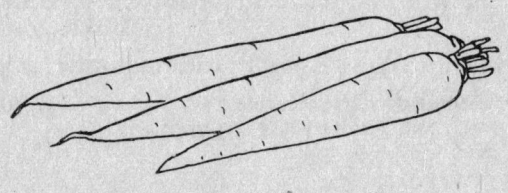

CLASSIC PILAF

 1 small onion, chopped
 1 tablespoon margarine
 1 cup UNCLE BEN'S® CONVERTED® Brand Rice
2½ cups chicken or beef broth

Cook onion in margarine in 10-inch skillet until tender but not brown. Add rice. Cook over low heat, stirring constantly, 5 minutes. Add chicken broth. Bring to a boil. Reduce heat. Cover tightly and simmer 20 minutes. Remove from heat. Let stand covered until all liquid is absorbed, about 5 minutes.

Makes 6 servings

Per Serving: *145 calories, 3 g protein, 2 g fat, 27 g carbohydrate, 327 mg sodium*

CHARLESTON RICE

½ cup each: coarsely chopped onion, celery, green pepper
1 tablespoon margarine
3 cups cooked rice*
1 can (2½ ounces) mushrooms, drained and chopped
½ teaspoon each: poultry seasoning, salt
¼ teaspoon each: celery seed, pepper
1 egg, beaten

Cook onion, celery and green pepper in margarine in skillet until tender. Add rice, mushrooms, poultry seasoning, salt, celery seed and pepper. Stir in egg. Spoon into lightly greased shallow 1½-quart casserole. Cover and bake at 350°F. for 15 minutes.

Makes 6 servings

*Cooked in chicken broth without butter or salt.

Per Serving: *125 calories, 3 g protein, 3 g fat, 21 g carbohydrate, 472 mg sodium*

BROWN RICE MEDLEY

2⅔ cups chicken broth
2 garlic cloves, minced
2 medium carrots, cut diagonally into ¼-inch slices
¼ teaspoon freshly ground pepper
1 cup UNCLE BEN'S® Select Brown Rice
1 cup thinly sliced mushrooms
¼ cup finely chopped green onions with tops

Combine chicken broth, garlic, carrots and pepper in medium saucepan. Bring to a boil. Add rice. Cover tightly and cook over low heat 45 minutes. Add mushrooms and green onions. Cover and continue cooking until all liquid is absorbed, about 5 minutes.

Makes 6 servings

Per Serving: *140 calories, 4 g protein, 1 g fat, 28 g carbohydrate, 336 mg sodium*

FIESTA THYME RICE

1 garlic clove, minced
2 teaspoons margarine
2½ cups water
1 cup UNCLE BEN'S® CONVERTED® Brand Rice
1 teaspoon salt
1 teaspoon dried thyme
1 tomato, chopped
4 green onions with tops, sliced

Cook garlic in margarine in medium saucepan 2 to 3 minutes. Add water and bring to a boil. Stir in rice, salt and thyme. Cover tightly and simmer 20 minutes. Remove from heat. Stir in tomato and green onions. Let stand covered until all water is absorbed, about 5 minutes.

Makes 6 servings

Per Serving: *135 calories, 2 g protein, 1 g fat, 27 g carbohydrate, 370 mg sodium*

Side Dishes

RISOTTO ALLA NAPOLITANA

- 1 can (8¼ ounces) whole tomatoes
- 1 can (13¾ or 14½ ounces) beef broth
- 1 large onion, chopped
- 1 garlic clove, minced
- 1½ tablespoons margarine
- 1 cup UNCLE BEN'S® CONVERTED® Brand Rice
- ½ teaspoon dried basil, crushed
- ⅛ teaspoon pepper
- 2 tablespoons grated Parmesan cheese

Drain and coarsely chop tomatoes, reserving liquid. Combine liquid and beef broth. Add water, if needed, to equal 2½ cups; set aside. Cook onion and garlic in margarine in large saucepan over low heat until onion is tender. Add rice. Cook, stirring constantly, 4 to 5 minutes. Add liquid, tomatoes, basil and pepper. Bring to a boil. Reduce heat. Cover tightly and simmer 20 minutes. Remove from heat. Let stand covered until all liquid is absorbed, about 5 minutes. Sprinkle with cheese. Stir lightly with fork.

Makes 6 servings

Per Serving: *180 calories, 5 g protein, 4 g fat, 30 g carbohydrate, 343 mg sodium*

PARMESAN EGGPLANT SKILLET

- 1 cup UNCLE BEN'S® CONVERTED® Brand Rice
- 1 tablespoon olive oil
- 2 medium onions, sliced
- 2 garlic cloves, minced
- ½ small eggplant (about ½ pound), cut into chunks
- 2 medium tomatoes, chopped
- 1 teaspoon salt
- 1 teaspoon dried oregano, crushed
- 2 tablespoons grated Parmesan cheese

Prepare rice according to package directions omitting butter and salt. Meanwhile, heat oil in 10-inch non-stick skillet. Add onions and garlic. Cook over medium heat, stirring constantly, until onion is tender. Stir in eggplant. Cover tightly and cook until eggplant is almost tender, about 5 minutes. Stir in tomatoes, salt and oregano. Cover and cook until vegetables are tender, about 5 minutes. Uncover and continue cooking, allowing any excess moisture to evaporate. Stir in hot cooked rice. Sprinkle with cheese.
Makes 6 servings

Per Serving: 175 calories, 4 g protein, 3 g fat, 32 g carbohydrate, 395 mg sodium

CARIBBEAN ISLAND RICE

1 cup uncooked rice
1 cup orange juice
1 cup chicken broth
1 teaspoon salt (optional)
¼ teaspoon white pepper
¼ cup flaked or shredded coconut
1 tablespoon unsalted margarine
2 cups peeled and diced papaya or mango*

Combine rice, juice, chicken broth, salt, if desired, and pepper in medium saucepan. Bring to a boil; stir once or twice. Reduce heat. Cover and simmer 15 minutes, or until rice is tender and liquid is absorbed. Stir in coconut and margarine. Let stand covered 10 minutes. Fold in papaya.
Makes 6 servings

*2 cups diced mangos or peaches, packed in juice, drained, may be substituted.

Per Serving: 170 calories, 3 g protein, 3 g fat, 32 g carbohydrate, 107 mg sodium when prepared without salt

GREEN PEPPERS STUFFED WITH MEDITERRANEAN RICE

2½ cups water
1 cup UNCLE BEN'S® CONVERTED® Brand Rice
1 medium tomato, chopped
6 green onions with tops, chopped
⅓ cup chopped ripe olives
1 garlic clove, minced
1 tablespoon olive oil
½ teaspoon salt
3 large green peppers, cut in half lengthwise
3 tablespoons grated Parmesan cheese

Bring water to a boil in medium saucepan. Stir in rice. Cover tightly and simmer 20 minutes. Meanwhile, combine tomato, green onions, olives, garlic, oil and salt; cover and set aside. Parboil green pepper halves in small amount of boiling water 3 to 5 minutes. Drain well. Remove rice from heat. Let stand covered until all water is absorbed, about 5 minutes. Stir tomato mixture into rice. Fill pepper halves with rice mixture, using about ⅔ cup for each. Sprinkle with cheese.

Makes 6 servings

Per Serving: *175 calories, 4 g protein, 4 g fat, 30 g carbohydrate, 308 mg sodium*

WALDORF-STYLE RICE

¾ cup chopped onion
2 teaspoons margarine
2 cups apple juice
½ cup water
½ teaspoon salt
1 cup UNCLE BEN'S® CONVERTED® Brand Rice
2 medium tart red apples, chopped
¾ cup thinly sliced celery
¼ cup chopped walnuts

Cook onion in margarine in medium saucepan until tender but not brown. Add apple juice, water and salt. Bring to a boil. Stir in rice. Cover tightly and simmer 20 minutes. Stir in apples, celery and walnuts. Remove from heat. Let stand covered until all liquid is absorbed, about 5 minutes.

Makes 8 servings

Per Serving: 180 calories, 3 g protein, 3 g fat, 34 g carbohydrate, 164 mg sodium

BROWN RICE GUADALAJARA

⅔ cup chopped onion
1 garlic clove, minced
2 teaspoons margarine
2⅔ cups water
1 cup UNCLE BEN'S® Select Brown Rice
1 teaspoon salt (optional)
3 ears sweet corn*
1 can (4 ounces) chopped green chilies, drained
1 teaspoon ground cumin
1 large tomato, cut into ½-inch pieces
2 tablespoons finely chopped parsley

Cook onion and garlic in margarine in medium saucepan until onion is tender but not brown. Add water and bring to a boil. Stir in rice and, if desired, salt. Cover tightly and cook over low heat 45 minutes. Cut corn kernels from cobs with sharp knife. Stir corn, chilies and cumin into rice. Cover and continue cooking over low heat until all water is absorbed, about 5 minutes. Stir in tomato and parsley.

Makes 6 servings

*1 cup frozen corn, thawed and drained, may be substituted.

Per Serving: 180 calories, 4 g protein, 2 g fat, 36 g carbohydrate, 377 mg sodium when prepared with salt

TOMATO RICE RING ITALIAN-STYLE

   1 large tomato, thinly sliced crosswise
   1 cup UNCLE BEN'S® CONVERTED® Brand Rice
   1 tablespoon vegetable oil
   ½ pound green beans, cut into 1-inch pieces
   1 medium onion, chopped
   1 garlic clove, minced
   2 medium zucchini, cut into ¼-inch slices
   2 medium yellow squash, cut into ¼-inch slices
   ¾ teaspoon salt
   ½ teaspoon dried oregano, crushed
   2 teaspoons margarine
   2 tablespoons grated Parmesan cheese

Coat a 4½-cup ring mold with vegetable oil cooking spray. Line bottom with tomato slices. Prepare rice according to package directions omitting butter. While rice is cooking, heat oil in large non-stick skillet. Add green beans, onion and garlic. Cover and cook over low heat, stirring occasionally, 10 minutes. Add zucchini, yellow squash, salt and oregano. Cover and continue cooking until vegetables are just tender, about 10 minutes. Remove from heat; stir in margarine. Stir cheese into rice. Lightly spoon rice mixture into prepared mold. Let stand about 5 minutes. Turn out onto serving platter. Fill center with vegetables.

Makes 8 servings

Per Serving: *150 calories, 4 g protein, 3 g fat, 26 g carbohydrate, 507 mg sodium*

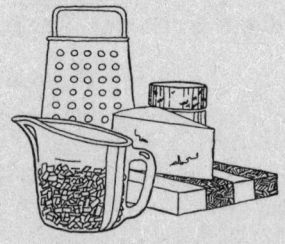

RISOTTO ALLA MILANESE

   Dash saffron (optional)
2½ cups beef broth or bouillon
  1 medium onion, chopped
  1 garlic clove, minced
  1 tablespoon margarine
  1 cup UNCLE BEN'S® CONVERTED® Brand Rice
  2 tablespoons dry sherry
  3 tablespoons grated Parmesan cheese

Stir saffron, if desired, into broth; set aside. Cook onion and garlic in margarine in 10-inch non-stick skillet over low heat until onion is tender. Add rice. Cook, stirring constantly, 4 to 5 minutes. Add broth and sherry. Bring to a boil. Reduce heat. Cover tightly and simmer 20 minutes. Remove from heat. Let stand covered until all liquid is absorbed, about 5 minutes. Sprinkle with cheese. Stir lightly with fork.

Makes 6 servings

Per Serving: *165 calories, 6 g protein, 3 g fat, 28 g carbohydrate, 400 mg sodium*

BROWN RICE ROYAL

  2 cups sliced mushrooms
  ½ cup finely chopped green onions with tops
  2 tablespoons vegetable oil
  3 cups cooked brown rice*

Cook mushrooms and onions in oil in large skillet until tender. Add rice; toss lightly. Heat through.

Makes 6 servings

*Cooked in beef broth without butter or salt.

Per Serving: *145 calories, 3 g protein, 5 g fat, 21 g carbohydrate, 364 mg sodium*

APRICOT BROWN RICE

 1 can (16 or 17 ounces) unpeeled apricot halves, packed in juice
2⅔ cups water
 1 cup UNCLE BEN'S® Select Brown Rice
 2 teaspoons margarine
 1 teaspoon salt (optional)
 ½ to 1 teaspoon finely chopped fresh ginger
 ⅓ cup coarsely chopped cashews

Drain apricots. Chop enough apricots to yield ½ cup; reserve remaining halves. Bring water to a boil in medium saucepan. Stir in rice, margarine and, if desired, salt. Cover tightly and cook over low heat 45 minutes. Stir in chopped apricots and ginger. Cover and continue cooking until all liquid is absorbed, about 5 minutes. Garnish each serving with cashews and reserved apricot halves.

Makes 6 servings

Per Serving: 175 calories, 3 g protein, 5 g fat, 29 g carbohydrate, 374 mg sodium when prepared with salt

BROCCOLI RICE WITH TOASTED WALNUTS

 1 cup UNCLE BEN'S® CONVERTED® Brand Rice
 1 pound broccoli (1 small bunch)
 1 tablespoon soy sauce
 1 tablespoon dry sherry
 1 tablespoon water
 1 teaspoon sugar
 1 tablespoon vegetable oil
 1 garlic clove, sliced
 ⅓ cup coarsely chopped walnuts

Prepare rice according to package directions omitting butter. Meanwhile, cut broccoli from stems into small flowerets, cutting any large ones in half.

Cut stems into thin strips, about 3 inches long. Combine soy sauce, sherry, water and sugar; mix well. Heat oil in 10-inch non-stick skillet. Add garlic and brown lightly. Remove garlic and discard. Add walnuts to skillet and brown lightly. Remove and set aside. Add broccoli. Cook and stir over medium heat until hot but not browned, 2 to 3 minutes. Stir in soy mixture. Cover and continue cooking until broccoli is tender, 2 to 4 minutes. Stir in hot cooked rice. Sprinkle with toasted walnuts.

Makes 8 servings

Per Serving: 165 calories, 5 g protein, 5 g fat, 24 g carbohydrate, 406 mg sodium

COUNTRY BREAKFAST CEREAL

2¼ cups water
1 cup uncooked brown rice
½ cup chopped prunes or raisins
1 tablespoon margarine
1 teaspoon ground cinnamon

Combine all ingredients in 2-quart saucepan with tight-fitting lid. Bring to a boil; stir once or twice. Reduce heat. Cover and simmer 45 to 55 minutes or until rice is tender and liquid is absorbed. Fluff with fork. Serve with skim milk, honey or brown sugar, and fresh fruit, if desired.

Makes 6 servings

MICROWAVE INSTRUCTIONS: Combine all ingredients in microproof baking dish. Cover and cook on HIGH (maximum power) 5 minutes or until boiling. Reduce setting to 30% power and cook 45 to 55 minutes. Fluff with fork.

Per Serving: 175 calories, 3 g protein, 3 g fat, 33 g carbohydrate, 24 mg sodium when served without toppings

GREEN RICE

1¾ cups water
5 ounces frozen chopped spinach, thawed (half of a 10-ounce package)
2 tablespoons chopped onion
1 teaspoon margarine
1 teaspoon salt
Dash pepper
Garlic powder, to taste (optional)
⅔ cup UNCLE BEN'S® CONVERTED® Brand Rice

Combine water, spinach, onion, margarine, salt, pepper and, if desired, garlic powder in medium saucepan. Bring to a boil. Stir in rice. Cover tightly and simmer 20 minutes. Remove from heat. Let stand covered until all liquid is absorbed, about 5 minutes.

Makes 4 servings

Per Serving: 130 calories, 3 g protein, 1 g fat, 27 g carbohydrate, 574 mg sodium

RISOTTO WITH GARDEN VEGETABLES

1 can (13¾ or 14½ ounces) chicken broth
1 cup UNCLE BEN'S® CONVERTED® Brand Rice
1 onion, chopped
2 tablespoons vegetable oil
½ teaspoon salt
¼ pound green beans, cut into 1-inch pieces
½ pound mushrooms, sliced
1 can (14 ounces) artichoke hearts
Pepper, as desired
2 tablespoons grated Parmesan cheese

Add water to chicken broth to equal 2½ cups; set aside. Cook rice and onion in 1 tablespoon of the oil in medium saucepan over low heat until onion

is tender. Add liquid and salt. Bring to a boil.
Reduce heat. Cover tightly and simmer 20 minutes.
Remove from heat. Let stand covered until all liquid
is absorbed, about 5 minutes. While rice is cooking,
cook green beans in remaining 1 tablespoon oil in
10-inch non-stick skillet until crisp-tender. Remove
and set aside. Add mushrooms to skillet and cook
until tender. Drain and coarsely chop artichoke
hearts. Add artichokes and green beans to
mushrooms in skillet. Stir in hot cooked rice.
Season to taste with pepper. Sprinkle with cheese.
Makes 8 servings

*Per Serving: 160 calories, 5 g protein, 4 g fat,
26 g carbohydrate, 343 mg sodium*

SOUTHWESTERN RICE

1 tablespoon margarine
1 cup UNCLE BEN'S® CONVERTED® Brand Rice
⅓ cup chopped onion
¼ cup diced green chilies
1 can (10½ ounces) condensed beef broth
1 teaspoon Worcestershire sauce
¾ teaspoon cumin seeds
¼ cup chopped ripe olives

Melt margarine in medium saucepan. Add rice,
onion and chilies. Cook, stirring frequently, until
rice is lightly browned. Add enough water to broth
to equal 2½ cups. Add to saucepan with
Worcestershire sauce and cumin. Bring to a boil.
Reduce heat. Cover tightly and simmer 20 minutes.
Remove from heat. Let stand covered until all liquid
is absorbed, about 5 minutes. Stir in olives.
Makes 6 servings

*Per Serving: 155 calories, 4 g protein, 3 g fat,
28 g carbohydrate, 401 mg sodium*

HERBED VEGETABLE RICE

1 can (13¾ or 14½ ounces) chicken broth
1 cup UNCLE BEN'S® CONVERTED® Brand Rice
½ cup chopped onion
1 teaspoon margarine
½ teaspoon salt (optional)
Dash red pepper flakes
1 cup fresh corn kernels*
¼ cup chopped parsley
1 teaspoon dried basil, crushed
1 small red or green pepper, cut into julienne strips

Add enough water to chicken broth to equal 2½ cups. Bring to a boil in medium saucepan. Stir in rice, onion, margarine, salt, if desired, and red pepper flakes. Cover tightly and simmer 15 minutes. Stir in corn. Cover and continue simmering 5 minutes. Remove from heat. Let stand covered until all liquid is absorbed, about 5 minutes. Stir in parsley and basil. Sprinkle with red pepper strips.

Makes 6 servings

*1 cup frozen whole kernel corn, thawed and drained, or 1 can (about 8 ounces) whole kernel corn, drained, may be substituted.

Per Serving: 165 calories, 5 g protein, 1 g fat, 33 g carbohydrate, 391 mg sodium when prepared with salt

ALOHA RICE MEDLEY

1 can (20 ounces) pineapple chunks, packed in juice
1 cup UNCLE BEN'S® CONVERTED® Brand Rice
1 tablespoon margarine
1 teaspoon salt (optional)
¼ cup toasted coconut

Side Dishes

Drain pineapple, reserving juice. Add enough water to juice to equal 2½ cups. Bring to a boil in medium saucepan. Stir in rice, margarine and, if desired, salt. Cover tightly and simmer 20 minutes. Stir in pineapple. Remove from heat. Let stand covered until all liquid is absorbed, about 5 minutes. Sprinkle with coconut.

Makes 8 servings

Per Serving: 160 calories, 2 g protein, 2 g fat, 33 g carbohydrate, 287 mg sodium when prepared with salt

CALIFORNIA ALMOND PILAF

- 2 cups water
- 1 cup uncooked brown rice
- ¼ cup raisins
- 1 tablespoon instant minced onion
- 1 tablespoon chicken bouillon granules
- 1 tablespoon margarine
- ¼ teaspoon white pepper
- ⅓ cup toasted slivered almonds

Combine all ingredients except almonds in 2-quart saucepan. Bring to a boil; stir once or twice. Reduce heat. Cover and simmer 45 to 50 minutes or until rice is tender and liquid is absorbed. Remove from heat. Add almonds and fluff with fork.

Makes 8 servings

MICROWAVE INSTRUCTIONS: Combine all ingredients except almonds in microproof baking dish. Cover and cook on HIGH (maximum power) 5 minutes or until boiling. Reduce setting to 30% power and cook 45 to 55 minutes. Add almonds and fluff with fork.

Per Serving: 150 calories, 3 g protein, 5 g fat, 23 g carbohydrate, 601 mg sodium

SESAME ZUCCHINI RICE

- 1 tablespoon margarine
- 1 cup UNCLE BEN'S® CONVERTED® Brand Rice
- 3 tablespoons sesame seeds
- 1 can (13¾ or 14½ ounces) chicken broth
- 1 teaspoon salt (optional)
- ¼ teaspoon ground ginger
- 4 medium zucchini (about ¼ pound each), cut into 2½×¼×¼-inch strips
- 2 to 3 teaspoons soy sauce

Melt margarine in 10-inch skillet. Add rice and sesame seeds. Cook and stir over low heat until lightly browned. Add enough water to chicken broth to equal 2½ cups. Add to skillet with salt, if desired, and ginger. Bring to a boil. Reduce heat. Cover tightly and simmer 20 minutes. Add zucchini. Cover and continue cooking until liquid is absorbed and zucchini is crisp-tender, about 5 minutes. Stir in soy sauce.

Makes 6 servings

Per Serving: *180 calories, 5 g protein, 4 g fat, 30 g carbohydrate, 703 mg sodium when prepared with salt and 2 teaspoons soy sauce*

GRECIAN SPINACH RICE

- 1 medium onion, chopped
- 1 tablespoon olive oil or vegetable oil
- 2½ cups water
- 1 cup UNCLE BEN'S® CONVERTED® Brand Rice
- 1 tablespoon lemon juice
- 1 teaspoon salt
- ½ teaspoon garlic powder
- ½ teaspoon grated lemon peel
- 2 cups firmly packed fresh spinach leaves, coarsely chopped
- 1 medium tomato, chopped
- ⅓ cup crumbled feta cheese (optional)

Cook onion in oil in large saucepan until tender but not brown. Add water and bring to a boil. Stir in rice, lemon juice, salt, garlic powder and lemon peel. Cover tightly and simmer 20 minutes. Stir in spinach. Remove from heat. Let stand covered until all liquid is absorbed, about 5 minutes. Stir in tomato and, if desired, sprinkle with cheese.

Makes 6 servings

Per Serving: *150 calories, 3 g protein, 2 g fat, 29 g carbohydrate, 373 mg sodium when prepared without cheese*

GARDEN VEGETABLE PILAF

- 1 medium onion, chopped
- 2 garlic cloves, minced
- 1 tablespoon olive oil
- 1 cup UNCLE BEN'S® Select Brown Rice
- 1 can (13¾ or 14½ ounces) chicken broth
- 1 teaspoon dried basil, crushed
- 1 medium zucchini, cut into 1×¼×¼-inch strips
- 1 red or green pepper, cut into ½-inch pieces
- 1 tomato, coarsely chopped
- 2 tablespoons grated Parmesan cheese

Cook onion and garlic in oil in medium saucepan over low heat until onion is tender but not brown. Add rice. Cook over low heat, stirring constantly, until rice is lightly browned, about 5 minutes. Add enough water to chicken broth to equal 2⅔ cups. Add to saucepan with basil and bring to a boil. Cover tightly and cook over low heat 45 minutes. Add zucchini and red pepper. Cover and continue cooking until all liquid is absorbed, about 5 minutes. Stir in tomato. Sprinkle each serving with cheese.

Makes 6 servings

Per Serving: *170 calories, 5 g protein, 3 g fat, 29 g carbohydrate, 245 mg sodium*

BROWN RICE O'BRIEN

- 1 cup chopped green onions with tops
- 1/2 cup chopped green pepper
- 2 tablespoons vegetable oil
- 3 cups hot cooked brown rice*
- 3 tablespoons chopped pimientos
- Dash pepper

Cook onions and green pepper in oil in large skillet until crisp-tender. Add rice, pimientos and pepper; toss lightly. Heat through.

Makes 6 servings

*Cooked in beef broth without butter or salt.

Per Serving: *170 calories, 3 g protein, 5 g fat, 27 g carbohydrate, 368 mg sodium*

WEST COAST RAISIN RICE

- 1/2 cup chopped onion
- 2 teaspoons margarine
- 2 1/2 cups chicken broth
- 3/4 teaspoon grated fresh ginger OR 1/4 teaspoon ground ginger
- 1/2 teaspoon salt
- 1 cup UNCLE BEN'S® CONVERTED® Brand Rice
- 1/3 cup chopped dried apricots
- 1/2 cup raisins
- 1/4 cup toasted slivered almonds

Cook onion in margarine in medium saucepan until tender but not brown. Add chicken broth, ginger and salt. Bring to a boil. Stir in rice and apricots. Cover tightly and simmer 20 minutes. Remove from heat. Stir in raisins. Let stand covered until all liquid is absorbed, about 5 minutes. Stir in almonds.

Makes 8 servings

Per Serving: *175 calories, 4 g protein, 3 g fat, 33 g carbohydrate, 375 mg sodium*

Salads

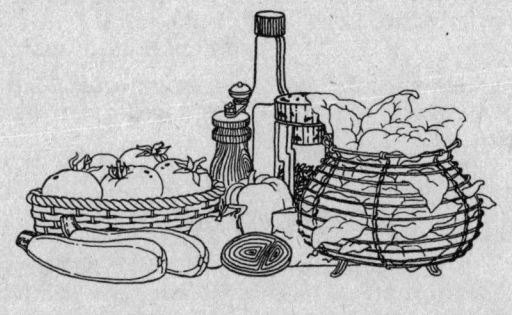

CURRIED CHICKEN SALAD

3⅓ cups water
1½ cups UNCLE BEN'S® CONVERTED® Brand Rice
2 cups diced cooked chicken
1 cup sliced celery
1 cup seedless grapes, halved
1 medium red or green pepper, cut into short thin strips
4 green onions with tops, thinly sliced
¾ cup reduced calorie mayonnaise
1½ tablespoons soy sauce
1 tablespoon curry powder
2 teaspoons lemon juice
1 teaspoon salt (optional)

Bring water to a boil in medium saucepan. Stir in rice. Cover tightly and simmer 20 minutes. Remove from heat. Let stand covered until all water is absorbed, about 5 minutes. Transfer to large bowl; cool to room temperature. Add chicken, celery, grapes, red pepper and green onions; mix well. Combine mayonnaise, soy sauce, curry powder, lemon juice and, if desired, salt. Stir dressing into rice mixture. Cover and chill several hours.
Makes 8 main dish servings

Per Serving: 285 calories, 14 g protein, 9 g fat, 36 g carbohydrate, 646 mg sodium when prepared with salt

ITALIAN RICE SALAD

1 cup UNCLE BEN'S® CONVERTED® Brand Rice
½ cup reduced calorie Italian-style salad dressing
2 tablespoons grated Parmesan cheese
Dash dried basil leaves, crushed
1 cup cooked and chilled peas
2 green onions with tops, sliced
¼ cup sliced ripe olives
2 tablespoons sliced pimiento

Prepare rice according to package directions omitting butter and salt. Transfer to large bowl. Cover and chill. Combine dressing, cheese and basil. Add to rice with remaining ingredients; mix well.

Makes 8 servings

Per Serving: *125 calories, 3 g protein, 2 g fat, 23 g carbohydrate, 175 mg sodium*

GULF COAST SALAD

- 3 cups cooked rice*
- 1 pound cooked shrimp, peeled and deveined**
- 1 cup sliced celery
- ½ cup sliced green onions with tops
- ⅔ cup reduced calorie mayonnaise
- 2 tablespoons catsup
- 1 teaspoon lemon juice
- ½ teaspoon cream-style prepared horseradish
- ½ teaspoon prepared mustard
- ⅛ teaspoon hot pepper sauce
- Salt (optional)
- White or black pepper
- Salad greens, as desired

Combine rice, shrimp, celery and green onions in large bowl. Stir together mayonnaise, catsup, lemon juice, horseradish, mustard and hot pepper sauce. Add to rice mixture; toss lightly. Season to taste with salt, if desired, and pepper. Cover and chill. Serve on salad greens.

Makes 6 main dish servings

*Cooked in chicken broth without butter or salt.

**If shrimp are large, cut in half lengthwise.

Per Serving: *270 calories, 16 g protein, 10 g fat, 28 g carbohydrate, 571 mg sodium when prepared without salt*

NICOISE RICE SALAD

- 2½ cups water
- 1 cup UNCLE BEN'S® CONVERTED® Brand Rice
- ⅓ cup olive oil
- 2 tablespoons vinegar
- 1 teaspoon dried basil, crushed
- 1 teaspoon salt
- ½ teaspoon freshly ground pepper
- 2 garlic cloves, minced
- 1 can (6½ or 7 ounces) tuna, packed in water, drained and flaked
- 1 cup cooked and chilled cut green beans
- ½ cup coarsely chopped ripe olives
- ½ cup julienne celery strips
- 6 green onions with tops, cut into 1-inch pieces
- ½ small green pepper, chopped
- 6 anchovies, chopped (optional)
- Salad greens, as desired
- 2 hard-cooked eggs, chopped
- 2 medium tomatoes, each cut into 6 wedges

Bring water to a boil in medium saucepan. Stir in rice. Cover tightly and simmer 20 minutes. Remove from heat. Let stand covered until all water is absorbed, about 5 minutes. Transfer to large bowl. Combine oil, vinegar, basil, salt, pepper and garlic. Add to hot rice; mix well. Cover and chill. Just before serving, add tuna, beans, olives, celery, onions, green pepper and, if desired, anchovies; toss lightly. Serve on salad greens garnished with eggs and tomato wedges.

Makes 6 main dish servings

Per Serving: *325 calories, 14 g protein, 15 g fat, 32 g carbohydrate, 498 mg sodium when prepared without anchovies*

ORIENTAL CHICKEN SALAD

- 2⅔ cups water
- 1 cup UNCLE BEN'S® Select Brown Rice
- 1 teaspoon salt (optional)
- 3 tablespoons vegetable oil
- 2 tablespoons white wine vinegar
- 2 tablespoons soy sauce
- 2 garlic cloves, minced
- 1½ cups diced cooked chicken
- 6 ounces fresh pea pods (cooked crisp-tender, if desired)*
- ¼ cup finely chopped green onions with tops
- 1 small red or green pepper, cut into short thin strips
- 1 teaspoon sesame oil (optional)

Bring water to a boil in medium saucepan. Add rice and, if desired, salt. Cover tightly and cook over low heat until all water is absorbed, about 50 minutes. Transfer to large bowl. Combine oil, vinegar, soy sauce and garlic. Add to hot rice with chicken. Cover and chill. Just before serving, stir in pea pods, onion, red pepper and, if desired, sesame oil.

Makes 6 main dish servings

*1 package (6 ounces) frozen pea pods, thawed and drained, may be substituted.

Per Serving: 255 calories, 15 g protein, 9 g fat, 28 g carbohydrate, 731 mg sodium when prepared with salt and without sesame oil

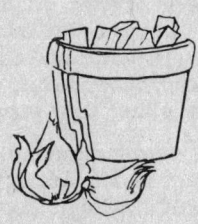

SUNSHINE RICE SALAD

- 1 cup UNCLE BEN'S® CONVERTED® Brand Rice
- ½ cup orange juice
- ⅓ cup reduced calorie Italian-style salad dressing
- 1 tablespoon honey
- 1 teaspoon grated orange peel
- 1 cup sliced celery
- 1 can (11 ounces) mandarin orange segments, drained
- ½ cup chopped red onion

Prepare rice according to package directions omitting butter and salt. Transfer to large bowl. Combine orange juice, dressing, honey and grated orange peel. Stir into hot cooked rice. Cover and chill. Just before serving, stir in remaining ingredients.

Makes 8 servings

Per Serving: 140 calories, 2 g protein, 1 g fat, 30 g carbohydrate, 103 mg sodium

GARDEN VEGETABLE RICE SALAD

- 2 cups water
- 1 cup uncooked rice
- 1 tablespoon margarine
- 1 teaspoon salt
- ½ teaspoon curry powder
- 1 medium tomato, coarsely chopped
- 1 medium carrot, diced
- ½ medium green pepper, cut into thin strips
- ½ medium red pepper, cut into thin strips
- ¼ cup oil and vinegar salad dressing
- ¼ teaspoon hot pepper sauce
- ½ small onion, sliced and separated into rings

Combine water, rice, margarine, salt and curry powder in 2-quart saucepan. Bring to a boil; stir once or twice. Reduce heat. Cover and simmer 15 minutes or until rice is tender and liquid is absorbed. Transfer rice to large bowl; cool to room temperature. Add tomato, carrot and green and red peppers. Combine dressing and hot pepper sauce. Pour over rice mixture; toss lightly. Garnish with onion rings.

Makes 6 servings

Per Serving: 210 calories, 3 g protein, 8 g fat, 31 g carbohydrate, 647 mg sodium

BROWN RICE CHEF'S SALAD BOWL

2⅔ cups water
1 cup UNCLE BEN'S® Select Brown Rice
1½ cups broccoli flowerets
½ pound mushrooms, sliced
1 cup cooked turkey breast strips, about 1×¼×¼ inches
1 cup (4 ounces) low-moisture, part-skim mozzarella cheese strips, about 1×¼×¼ inches
½ cup reduced calorie mayonnaise
2 tablespoons vinegar
1 tablespoon Dijon-style mustard
1 teaspoon salt
½ teaspoon sugar
¼ teaspoon pepper

Bring water to a boil in medium saucepan. Stir in rice. Cover tightly and cook over low heat until all water is absorbed, about 50 minutes. Transfer rice to large bowl; cool to room temperature. Add broccoli, mushrooms, turkey and cheese. Place remaining ingredients in blender container or jar with tight-fitting lid; cover and blend. Add to rice; mix well. Cover and chill at least two hours.

Makes 6 main dish servings

Per Serving: 285 calories, 16 g protein, 11 g fat, 30 g carbohydrate, 635 mg sodium

VEGETABLE MEDLEY SALAD WITH SHERRY DRESSING

3⅓ cups water
1½ cups UNCLE BEN'S® CONVERTED® Brand Rice
1½ teaspoons salt
 2 medium carrots, sliced diagonally
 ½ cup vegetable oil
 ¼ cup dry sherry
 1 small yellow squash, cut into 1×¼×¼-inch strips
 1 cup small broccoli flowerets
 8 to 10 cherry tomatoes, cut in half
 ½ cup sliced radishes
 ¼ cup cider vinegar
 1 garlic clove, minced
 1 teaspoon sugar

Bring water to a boil in medium saucepan. Stir in rice and salt. Cover tightly and simmer 20 minutes. Remove from heat. Let stand covered until all water is absorbed, about 5 minutes. Transfer to large bowl; cool to room temperature. Cook carrots in 1 tablespoon of the oil and 1 tablespoon of the sherry, in skillet, 1 to 2 minutes. Add squash and broccoli. Cook until vegetables are crisp-tender, about 1 minute. Add to rice with tomatoes and radishes. Combine remaining oil and sherry, vinegar, garlic and sugar. Add to rice; mix well. Cover and chill several hours.

Makes 10 servings

Per Serving: *220 calories, 3 g protein, 11 g fat, 27 g carbohydrate, 333 mg sodium*

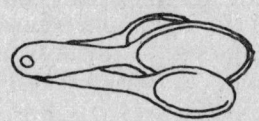

PEPPERY BROWN RICE & TOMATO SALAD

2⅔ cups water
1 cup UNCLE BEN'S® Select Brown Rice
2 medium tomatoes, cut into ½-inch pieces
⅓ cup reduced calorie mayonnaise
1 tablespoon lemon juice
1 teaspoon salt
1 to 2 garlic cloves
¼ to ½ teaspoon hot pepper sauce
⅛ to ¼ teaspoon pepper
1 small cucumber

Bring water to a boil in medium saucepan. Stir in rice. Cover tightly and cook over low heat until all water is absorbed, about 50 minutes. Transfer to large bowl; cool to room temperature. Combine ½ cup of the tomato pieces, mayonnaise, lemon juice, salt, garlic, hot pepper sauce and pepper in blender or food processor container. Blend until smooth, 1 to 2 minutes. Stir dressing into rice. Cover and chill several hours or overnight. Cover and refrigerate remaining tomato pieces. Just before serving, slice cucumber ¼ inch thick; cut each slice in half. Add cucumber and reserved tomato pieces to rice; toss lightly.

Makes 6 servings

Per Serving: *170 calories, 3 g protein, 5 g fat, 28 g carbohydrate, 442 mg sodium*

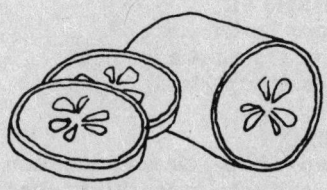

SWEET & SOUR TUNA SALAD

- 1 can (15½ ounces) pineapple chunks, packed in juice
- ½ cup reduced calorie mayonnaise
- 2 teaspoons soy sauce
- ½ teaspoon garlic salt
- 3½ cups cooked and chilled UNCLE BEN'S® CONVERTED® Brand Rice*
- 1 can (6½ or 7 ounces) tuna, packed in water, drained and flaked
- 1 small green pepper, cut into short thin strips
- 12 cherry tomatoes, halved
- Salad greens, as desired

Drain pineapple chunks, reserving 2 tablespoons juice. Combine juice, mayonnaise, soy sauce and garlic salt in large bowl; mix well. Stir in rice, tuna, green pepper and pineapple; mix lightly. Cover and chill. Just before serving, fold in cherry tomatoes. Serve on salad greens.

Makes 4 main dish servings

*Prepared without butter or salt.

Per Serving: 395 calories, 18 g protein, 11 g fat, 56 g carbohydrate, 513 mg sodium

CITRUSY BROWN RICE SHRIMP SALAD

- 2⅔ cups water
- 1 cup UNCLE BEN'S® Select Brown Rice
- ⅓ cup vegetable oil
- 2 tablespoons lemon juice
- 1 tablespoon grated orange peel
- 1 teaspoon salt (optional)
- ¼ teaspoon pepper
- 2 navel oranges
- ½ pound cooked and cleaned medium shrimp
- 3 green onions with tops, thinly sliced
- Salad greens (optional)

Bring water to a boil in medium saucepan. Stir in rice. Cover tightly and cook over low heat until all water is absorbed, about 50 minutes. Transfer to large bowl. Combine oil, lemon juice, orange peel, salt, if desired, and pepper. Stir into hot rice. Cover and chill at least 4 hours. Just before serving, peel and section oranges; cut each section in half. Stir oranges, shrimp and green onions into rice. Serve on salad greens, if desired.

Makes 6 main dish servings

Per Serving: *290 calories, 12 g protein, 13 g fat, 30 g carbohydrate, 359 mg sodium when prepared with salt and without salad greens*

RICE FONTINA SALAD

4 cups cooked and cooled rice*
1 cup (4 ounces) grated Fontina or Swiss cheese
1 small zucchini, cut into thin 1-inch strips
½ cup chopped celery
½ cup sliced ripe olives
¼ cup chopped onion
½ cup reduced calorie mayonnaise
½ cup plain yogurt
1 teaspoon white wine vinegar
½ teaspoon salt
¼ teaspoon dried basil leaves, crushed
¼ teaspoon dried oregano leaves, crushed
¼ teaspoon pepper
⅛ teaspoon garlic powder
12 cherry tomatoes, halved

Combine rice, cheese, zucchini, celery, olives and onion in large bowl. Stir together remaining ingredients except tomatoes. Add to rice; mix well. Fold in tomatoes. Cover and chill.

Makes 10 servings

*Prepared without butter or salt.

Per Serving: *205 calories, 5 g protein, 11 g fat, 21 g carbohydrate, 413 mg sodium*

CALICO VEGETABLE RICE SALAD

2½ cups water
1 tablespoon chicken bouillon granules
¾ teaspoon onion salt
½ teaspoon freshly ground pepper
¼ teaspoon dried thyme, crushed
¼ teaspoon turmeric
⅛ teaspoon ground cumin
1 cup UNCLE BEN'S® CONVERTED® Brand Rice
¼ cup reduced calorie Italian-style salad dressing
1 cup sliced celery
1 jar (4 ounces) pimiento, drained and sliced
⅓ cup sliced ripe olives
2 tablespoons minced chives
Salad greens, as desired
2 medium tomatoes, each cut into 6 wedges

Combine water, bouillon granules, onion salt, pepper, thyme, turmeric and cumin in medium saucepan. Bring to a boil. Stir in rice. Cover tightly and simmer 20 minutes. Remove from heat. Let stand covered until all liquid is absorbed, about 5 minutes. Transfer to large bowl; cool to room temperature. Add dressing, celery, pimiento, olives and chives; toss lightly. Cover and chill. Serve on salad greens garnished with tomato wedges.

Makes 6 servings

Per Serving: *160 calories, 4 g protein, 2 g fat, 31 g carbohydrate, 334 mg sodium*

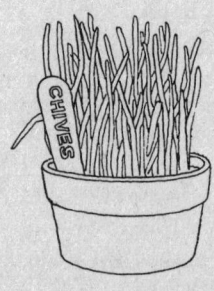

SPINACH SALAD WITH ORIENTAL VINAIGRETTE

- 2½ cups water
- 1 cup UNCLE BEN'S® CONVERTED® Brand Rice
- ⅓ cup olive oil
- 1 tablespoon vinegar
- 1 tablespoon soy sauce
- ½ teaspoon freshly ground pepper
- 2 garlic cloves, minced
- ¼ pound fresh spinach leaves, cut into julienne strips
- 4 green onions with tops, finely chopped
- 1 small zucchini, cut into julienne strips
- ½ cup julienne celery strips
- ⅓ cup toasted pine nuts or chopped walnuts
- Salad greens, as desired

Bring water to a boil in medium saucepan. Stir in rice. Cover tightly and simmer 20 minutes. Remove from heat. Let stand covered until all water is absorbed, about 5 minutes. Transfer to large bowl. Combine oil, vinegar, soy sauce, pepper and garlic. Add to hot rice; mix well. Cover and chill. Just before serving, add spinach, onions, zucchini, celery and pine nuts; toss lightly. Serve on salad greens.

Makes 8 servings

Per Serving: *215 calories, 4 g protein, 12 g fat, 23 g carbohydrate, 154 mg sodium*

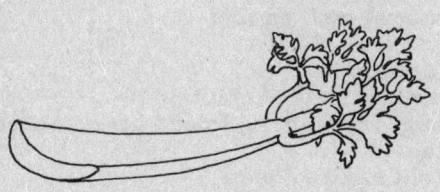

RICE SALAD MILANO

- 3 cups hot cooked rice*
- ¼ cup vegetable oil
- 2 tablespoons lemon juice
- 1 garlic clove, minced
- ½ teaspoon salt (optional)
- ½ teaspoon each: dried rosemary, dried oregano leaves
- ½ teaspoon pepper
- 1 small zucchini, thinly sliced
- 1 medium tomato, seeded and chopped
- 3 tablespoons grated Parmesan cheese

Spoon rice into large bowl. Combine oil, lemon juice, garlic, salt, if desired, rosemary, oregano and pepper. Stir into rice; cool to room temperature. Add remaining ingredients. Serve immediately or cover and chill.

Makes 8 servings

*Prepared without butter or salt.

Per Serving: 145 calories, 2 g protein, 8 g fat, 16 g carbohydrate, 22 mg sodium when prepared without salt

ARROZ CON POLLO SALAD

- 1 cup chopped onion
- ⅓ cup vegetable oil
- 2⅔ cups water
- 1 cup UNCLE BEN'S® Select Brown Rice
- 2 teaspoons chili powder
- 2 tablespoons vinegar
- 1 teaspoon salt
- 2 cups diced cooked chicken
- 1 package (10 ounces) frozen peas, cooked and drained
- ⅓ cup sliced ripe olives
- 1 medium tomato, chopped
- Salad greens, as desired

Cook onion in 2 teaspoons of the oil in medium saucepan until tender but not brown. Add water and bring to a boil. Stir in rice and chili powder. Cover tightly and cook over low heat until all liquid is absorbed, about 50 minutes. Transfer to large bowl. Combine remaining oil, the vinegar and salt. Add to hot rice with chicken, peas and olives. Cover and chill. Just before serving, stir in tomato. Serve on salad greens.

Makes 6 main dish servings

Per Serving: 370 calories, 20 g protein, 17 g fat, 34 g carbohydrate, 506 mg sodium when prepared without salad greens

BARBECUE BONUS SALAD

3½ cups cooked and chilled UNCLE BEN'S® CONVERTED® Brand Rice*
1 medium onion, minced
2 cups sliced celery
1 cup plain low-fat yogurt
¾ cup reduced calorie mayonnaise
4 teaspoons Dijon-style mustard
½ teaspoon salt
1 hard-cooked egg, chopped
½ cup sliced radishes
1 cucumber, diced
   Salad greens, as desired
1 large tomato, cut into wedges

Combine rice, onion and celery in large bowl. Combine yogurt, mayonnaise, mustard and salt. Add to rice mixture; mix well. Cover and chill. Just before serving, stir in egg, radishes and cucumber. Serve in bowl lined with salad greens garnished with tomato wedges.

Makes 8 servings

*Prepared without butter or salt.

Per Serving: 200 calories, 5 g protein, 9 g fat, 24 g carbohydrate, 375 mg sodium

CURRIED SUMMER FRUIT 'N BROWN RICE SALAD

2⅔ cups water
1 cup UNCLE BEN'S® Select Brown Rice
1 teaspoon curry powder
⅛ teaspoon ground cinnamon
½ cup plain low-fat yogurt
1 to 2 tablespoons honey
¼ teaspoon salt
2 ripe peaches or nectarines, peeled, if desired, and coarsely chopped*
2 cups cantaloupe or honeydew melon cubes (about 1 small melon)
1 cup seedless green grapes, halved if large
¼ cup toasted slivered almonds

Bring water to a boil in medium saucepan. Stir in rice, curry powder and cinnamon. Cover tightly and cook over low heat until all liquid is absorbed, about 50 minutes. Transfer to large bowl; cover and chill. Combine yogurt, honey and salt. Add to rice with fruits and almonds; mix well.

Makes 10 servings

*1 can (16 ounces) sliced peaches, packed in juice, chopped and drained, may be substituted.

Per Serving: *150 calories, 3 g protein, 3 g fat, 27 g carbohydrate, 68 mg sodium when prepared with 1 tablespoon honey*

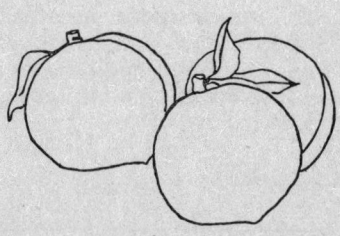

SPICY ORIENTAL RICE SALAD

2½ cups water
  1 cup UNCLE BEN'S® CONVERTED® Brand Rice
  1 teaspoon salt (optional)
  2 cups cut-up cooked chicken or turkey
  1 carrot, cut into 1×¼×¼-inch strips
  2 green onions with tops, sliced
  1 cup fresh pea pods, cut diagonally into 1-inch pieces and blanched*
  ¼ cup red wine vinegar
  3 tablespoons vegetable oil
  2 tablespoons soy sauce
  2 tablespoons honey
  2 teaspoons grated fresh ginger OR ½ teaspoon ground ginger
  ½ teaspoon crushed red pepper flakes
  1 garlic clove, minced

Bring water to a boil in medium saucepan. Stir in rice and, if desired, salt. Cover tightly and simmer 20 minutes. Remove from heat. Let stand covered until all water is absorbed, about 5 minutes. Transfer to large bowl; cool to room temperature. Add chicken, carrot, green onions and pea pods. Combine vinegar, oil, soy sauce, honey, ginger, red pepper flakes and garlic. Add to rice mixture; mix well. Cover and chill several hours.

Makes 6 main dish servings

*1 cup frozen pea pods, thawed, may be substituted.

Per Serving: *300 calories, 18 g protein, 9 g fat, 35 g carbohydrate, 744 mg sodium when prepared with salt*

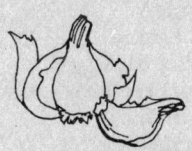

TUNA AND BROWN RICE SALAD

2⅔ cups water
 1 cup UNCLE BEN'S® Select Brown Rice
 ½ cup chopped onion
 1 teaspoon salt (optional)
 ½ cup reduced calorie Italian-style salad dressing
    Spinach leaves
 1 cup diced carrots
 1 can (6½ or 7 ounces) tuna, packed in water,
    drained and flaked
 3 tablespoons snipped parsley
    Freshly ground pepper
 1 large tomato, cut into wedges

Bring water to a boil in medium saucepan. Add rice, onion and, if desired, salt. Cover tightly and cook over low heat until all water is absorbed, about 50 minutes. Transfer to large bowl. Stir in dressing; cover and chill. At serving time, arrange spinach leaves on individual salad plates. Stir carrots, tuna and parsley into rice. Spoon about ¾ cup rice mixture onto each plate. Sprinkle with pepper and garnish with tomato wedges.

Makes 6 main dish servings

Per Serving: *210 calories, 13 g protein, 3 g fat, 32 g carbohydrate, 566 mg sodium when prepared with salt*

SUMMER'S SPECIAL BROWN RICE FRUIT SALAD

2⅔ cups water
 1 cup UNCLE BEN'S® Select Brown Rice
 ¼ cup lemon juice
 3 tablespoons honey
 1 tablespoon dry sherry
 2 peaches or nectarines, coarsely chopped
 1 cup blueberries
 1 cup sliced strawberries

Bring water to a boil in medium saucepan. Stir in rice. Cover tightly and cook over low heat until all water is absorbed, about 50 minutes. Transfer to large bowl; cover and chill. Combine lemon juice, honey and sherry. Add to rice with fruit; toss lightly.

Makes 10 servings

Per Serving: *115 calories, 2 g protein, less than 1 g fat, 25 g carbohydrate, 3 mg sodium*

JAMBALAYA RICE SALAD

2½ cups water
1 cup UNCLE BEN'S® CONVERTED® Brand Rice
1 teaspoon salt
½ teaspoon hot pepper sauce
¼ cup vegetable oil
2 tablespoons red wine vinegar
1 garlic clove, minced
½ pound cooked and cleaned medium shrimp
¾ cup diced cooked ham
4 green onions with tops, sliced
1 small green pepper, cut into 1×¼×¼-inch strips
2 medium tomatoes, coarsely chopped

Bring water to a boil in medium saucepan. Stir in rice, ½ teaspoon of the salt and the hot pepper sauce. Cover tightly and simmer 20 minutes. Remove from heat. Let stand covered until all liquid is absorbed, about 5 minutes. Transfer to large bowl. Combine oil, vinegar, remaining ½ teaspoon salt and the garlic. Add to rice with shrimp, ham, onions and green pepper; mix well. Cover and chill at least 3 hours. Stir in tomatoes.

Makes 6 main dish servings

Per Serving: *285 calories, 15 g protein, 12 g fat, 29 g carbohydrate, 642 mg sodium*

SEAFOOD SALAD WITH ORANGE VINAIGRETTE

2½ cups water
1 cup UNCLE BEN'S® CONVERTED® Brand Rice
⅓ cup olive oil
2 tablespoons lemon juice
2 tablespoons grated orange peel
¾ teaspoon salt
½ teaspoon freshly ground pepper
½ pound cooked and cleaned medium shrimp, chilled
½ pound cooked and chilled crabmeat
½ pound cooked and chilled bay scallops
½ cup diced red pepper
2 tablespoons chopped green chilies
2 green onions with tops, thinly sliced
Salad greens, as desired

Bring water to a boil in medium saucepan. Stir in rice. Cover tightly and simmer 20 minutes. Remove from heat. Let stand covered until all water is absorbed, about 5 minutes. Transfer to large bowl. Combine oil, lemon juice, orange peel, salt and pepper. Add to hot rice; mix well. Cover and chill. Just before serving, add seafood, red pepper, chilies and green onions; toss lightly. Serve on salad greens.

Makes 8 main dish servings

Per Serving: *275 calories, 21 g protein, 11 g fat, 22 g carbohydrate, 600 mg sodium*

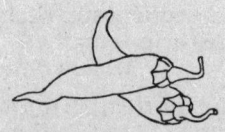

THREE MELON RICE SALAD

- 2½ cups water
- 1 cup UNCLE BEN'S® CONVERTED® Brand Rice
- 1 teaspoon salt
- ⅓ cup orange juice
- 2 tablespoons lemon juice
- 2 tablespoons sugar
- ¼ cup vegetable oil
- 1 teaspoon poppy seeds
- 1 teaspoon grated orange peel
- 1 teaspoon finely chopped fresh mint leaves OR ¼ teaspoon dried mint leaves
- 1 cup small watermelon balls
- 1 cup small honeydew melon balls
- 1 cup small cantaloupe balls

Bring water to a boil in medium saucepan. Stir in rice and salt. Cover tightly and simmer 20 minutes. Remove from heat. Let stand covered until all water is absorbed, about 5 minutes. Transfer to large bowl; cool to room temperature. Combine orange juice, lemon juice and sugar in blender or food processor container. Blend 1 to 2 minutes. Gradually add oil, blending until slightly thickened. Add poppy seeds, orange peel and mint; blend 10 seconds. Stir dressing into rice. Cover and chill several hours. Add melon balls; mix well.

Makes 8 servings

Per Serving: 185 calories, 2 g protein, 7 g fat, 28 g carbohydrate, 274 mg sodium

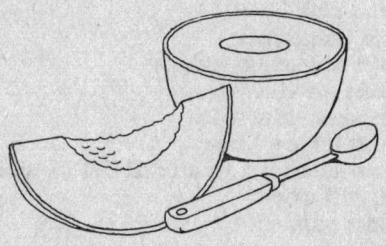

ARABIAN RICE SALAD

2⅔ cups water
1 cup UNCLE BEN'S® Select Brown Rice
¾ cup loosely packed minced parsley
½ cup loosely packed fresh mint leaves, chopped, OR 2 teaspoons dried mint leaves
4 green onions with tops, sliced
1 cup diced cucumber
3 medium tomatoes, diced
⅓ cup olive oil
¼ to ⅓ cup lemon juice
¾ teaspoon salt
½ teaspoon pepper
Spinach leaves (optional)

Bring water to a boil in medium saucepan. Stir in rice. Cover tightly and cook over low heat until all water is absorbed, about 50 minutes. Transfer to large bowl; cool to room temperature. Add parsley, mint, green onions, cucumber and tomatoes. Combine oil, lemon juice, salt and pepper. Add to rice mixture; mix well. Cover and chill. Serve on spinach leaves, if desired.

Makes 10 servings

Per Serving: 155 calories, 2 g protein, 8 g fat, 18 g carbohydrate, 272 mg sodium

DILLY CUCUMBER RICE SALAD

2½ cups water
1 cup UNCLE BEN'S® CONVERTED® Brand Rice
1 teaspoon salt
1 medium cucumber
½ cup thin red onion wedges
1 cup plain low-fat yogurt
2 tablespoons skim milk
1 teaspoon lemon juice
1 teaspoon chopped fresh dill OR ¼ teaspoon dried dill weed
¼ teaspoon pepper

Bring water to a boil in medium saucepan. Stir in rice and ½ teaspoon of the salt. Cover tightly and simmer 20 minutes. Remove from heat. Let stand covered until all water is absorbed, about 5 minutes. Transfer to large bowl; cool to room temperature. Slice cucumber into ¼-inch slices; cut each slice into quarters. Add cucumber and onion to rice. Combine yogurt, milk, lemon juice, dill, pepper and remaining ½ teaspoon salt. Stir dressing into rice mixture. Cover and chill several hours.

Makes 6 servings

Per Serving: 145 calories, 4 g protein, 1 g fat, 29 g carbohydrate, 379 mg sodium

HAWAIIAN TURKEY SALAD

- 1 can (8 ounces) pineapple chunks, packed in juice
- 3 cups cooked brown rice*
- 2 cups coarsely chopped cooked turkey
- 1 can (8 ounces) sliced water chestnuts, drained
- 1 medium unpeeled apple, chopped
- ⅓ cup chopped macadamia nuts
- ½ teaspoon salt
- ½ cup plain yogurt
  Lettuce leaves, as desired
- ¼ cup shredded coconut, toasted

Drain pineapple, reserving 1 tablespoon juice. Combine pineapple, rice, turkey, water chestnuts, apple, macadamia nuts and salt in large bowl. Stir together yogurt and reserved pineapple juice. Add to rice mixture; toss lightly. Serve on lettuce leaves garnished with coconut.

Makes 6 main dish servings

*Prepared without butter or salt.

Per Serving: 285 calories, 14 g protein, 10 g fat, 34 g carbohydrate, 223 mg sodium

MEAL-IN-ONE SALAD

3½ cups cooked and chilled UNCLE BEN'S® CONVERTED® Brand Rice*
½ pound fresh spinach, torn into bite-size pieces
¾ cup thinly sliced green onions with tops
¼ pound Canadian bacon, cut into thin strips
¼ pound Swiss cheese, cut into thin strips
½ cup thinly sliced radishes
1 teaspoon salt
1 teaspoon seasoned pepper
⅓ cup reduced calorie Italian-style salad dressing
  Salad greens, as desired
4 hard-cooked eggs, chopped

Combine rice, spinach, onions, Canadian bacon, Swiss cheese, radishes, salt and seasoned pepper in large bowl. Add dressing; toss lightly. Serve on salad greens garnished with eggs.

Makes 6 main dish servings

*Prepared without butter or salt.

Per Serving: 280 calories, 17 g protein, 12 g fat, 26 g carbohydrate, 853 mg sodium

RICE SALAD ITALIA

2½ cups water
1 cup UNCLE BEN'S® CONVERTED® Brand Rice
1½ teaspoons salt
½ pound cooked ham, cut into ¼-inch chunks
¼ pound mushrooms, sliced
½ cup pitted ripe olives, quartered
½ cup diced green pepper
⅓ cup vegetable oil
2 tablespoons cider vinegar
½ teaspoon dried basil, crushed
¼ teaspoon pepper
1 garlic clove, minced
1 medium tomato, coarsely chopped

Bring water to a boil in medium saucepan. Stir in rice and 1 teaspoon of the salt. Cover tightly and simmer 20 minutes. Remove from heat. Let stand covered until all water is absorbed, about 5 minutes. Transfer to large bowl; cool to room temperature. Add ham, mushrooms, olives and green pepper. Combine oil, vinegar, basil, pepper, garlic and remaining ½ teaspoon salt. Add to rice mixture; mix well. Cover and chill. Just before serving, stir in tomato.

Makes 6 main dish servings

Per Serving: 315 calories, 10 g protein, 17 g fat, 29 g carbohydrate, 1121 mg sodium

FRUIT-OF-THE-SEASON RICE SALAD

- 1 cup UNCLE BEN'S® CONVERTED® Brand Rice
- 1 carton (8 ounces) banana or peach flavored low-fat yogurt
- 1 tablespoon honey
- 1 ripe banana, sliced
- 2 cups diced or sliced fresh fruits and berries
- ¼ cup chopped pecans

Prepare rice according to package directions omitting butter and salt. Transfer to large bowl; cool slightly. Combine yogurt and honey. Stir into warm rice. Cover and chill. Just before serving, stir in fruits and pecans.

Makes 8 servings

Per Serving: 175 calories, 3 g protein, 3 g fat, 34 g carbohydrate, 18 mg sodium

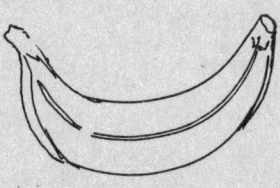

CHICKEN SALAD WITH TARRAGON VINAIGRETTE

2½ cups water
1 cup UNCLE BEN'S® CONVERTED® Brand Rice
⅓ cup olive oil
2 tablespoons lemon juice
1 teaspoon dried tarragon, crushed
1 teaspoon salt
½ teaspoon freshly ground pepper
2½ cups cooked chicken or turkey breast strips, about 1 × ¼ × ¼ inches
1 cup sliced celery
¼ cup toasted slivered almonds
¼ cup chopped parsley
Salad greens, as desired
1 large tomato, cut into wedges

Bring water to a boil in medium saucepan. Stir in rice. Cover tightly and simmer 20 minutes. Remove from heat. Let stand covered until all water is absorbed, about 5 minutes. Transfer to large bowl. Combine oil, lemon juice, tarragon, salt and pepper. Add to hot rice; mix well. Cover and chill. Just before serving, add chicken, celery, almonds and parsley; toss lightly. Serve on salad greens garnished with tomato wedges.

Makes 6 main dish servings

Per Serving: *375 calories, 22 g protein, 18 g fat, 30 g carbohydrate, 434 mg sodium*

Desserts

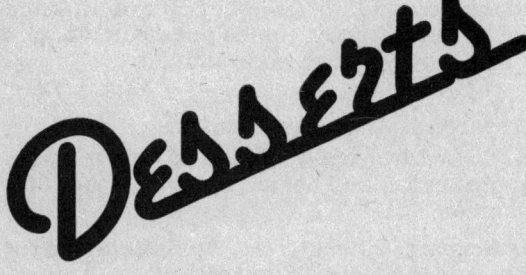
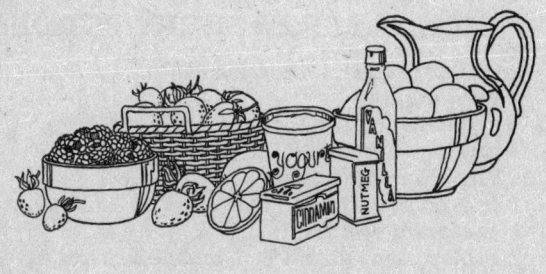

CITRUS RICE CHEESECAKE

3 eggs
1 cup sugar
1½ cups (15 ounces) ricotta cheese
½ cup 2 percent milk
2 teaspoons grated lemon or orange peel
5 cups cooked and cooled rice*

Beat together eggs and sugar about ½ minute. Add cheese, milk, and lemon peel; beat until well blended. Stir in rice. Pour into greased 9-inch square baking dish. Bake at 350°F. until knife inserted near center comes out clean, about 45 to 55 minutes. Serve warm or chilled.

Makes 12 servings

*Prepared without butter or salt.

NOTE: Leftover pudding may be covered with aluminum foil and heated at 250°F. about 30 minutes.

Per Serving: 225 calories, 7 g protein, 4 g fat, 40 g carbohydrate, 66 mg sodium

RICE 'N STRAWBERRY PUDDING

2 pints fresh strawberries
¾ cup sugar
1½ tablespoons lime juice
1 quart 2 percent milk
¾ cup uncooked rice
1 teaspoon salt
1 teaspoon vanilla
2 tablespoons rum OR 1 teaspoon rum extract (optional)

Reserve 8 strawberries for garnish. Slice remaining strawberries. Sprinkle with ¼ cup of the sugar and the lime juice; set aside. Bring milk, rice, salt and remaining ½ cup sugar to a boil in heavy saucepan with tight-fitting lid. Stir once or twice; reduce heat.

Cover and simmer 25 to 30 minutes, stirring occasionally, until rice is tender and milk is almost absorbed. Add vanilla and, if desired, rum. Transfer to large bowl; cool to room temperature. Fold in sliced strawberries. Spoon pudding into serving dishes. Serve immediately or cover and chill. Garnish with reserved whole berries.

Makes 8 servings

Per Serving: 220 calories, 5 g protein, 3 g fat, 42 g carbohydrate, 329 mg sodium

MAPLE WALNUT RICE CUSTARD

- 2 eggs
- 1⅓ cups skim milk
- 1 cup reduced calorie maple-flavored syrup
- 1½ cups cooked and cooled UNCLE BEN'S® CONVERTED® Brand Rice*
- 1 tablespoon margarine
- ¼ cup chopped walnuts

Combine eggs, milk and ½ cup of the syrup in bowl; mix well. Stir in rice. Pour into 1½-quart casserole. Place casserole in baking pan filled with 1 inch hot water. Bake at 350°F. about 1 hour and 15 minutes or until knife inserted 1 inch from center comes out clean. *Stir once after 30 minutes.* Remove pudding from oven. Cool on rack. Serve warm or chilled with warm Maple Topping.

Maple Topping: Combine remaining ½ cup syrup and the margarine in small saucepan. Cook over moderate heat, stirring constantly, until mixture comes to a boil. Reduce heat. Simmer 2 minutes, stirring constantly. Remove from heat. Stir in walnuts.

Makes 6 servings

*Prepared without butter or salt.

Per Serving: 170 calories, 6 g protein, 7 g fat, 20 g carbohydrate, 74 mg sodium

PINEAPPLE RICE BAKE

   3 cups cooked rice*
   3 cups 2 percent milk, divided
   ¼ cup sugar
   1 tablespoon margarine
   ½ teaspoon salt
   3 eggs, separated
   1 can (20 ounces) crushed pineapple, packed in juice
   1 teaspoon ground cinnamon

Combine rice, 2½ cups of the milk, the sugar, margarine and salt in medium saucepan. Cook over medium heat, stirring occasionally, until thick and creamy, about 25 minutes. Beat egg yolks. Combine yolks and remaining ½ cup milk; stir into rice. Cook and stir 2 minutes. Remove from heat. Stir in pineapple with juice and cinnamon. Cool. Beat egg whites until stiff but not dry. Fold into rice. Spoon into greased 9-inch square baking pan. Bake at 325°F. for 25 minutes or until knife inserted near center comes out clean.

Makes 8 servings

*Prepared without butter or salt.

Per Serving: 225 calories, 7 g protein, 5 g fat, 37 g carbohydrate, 226 mg sodium

FRUIT TREAT

2⅔ cups water
   1 cup UNCLE BEN'S® Select Brown Rice
   2 teaspoons margarine
   1 teaspoon salt (optional)
   ¼ cup honey
   ¼ cup lemon juice
   3 cups diced assorted fresh fruits and berries
   2 oranges, peeled, diced and drained
   1 large unpeeled Red Delicious apple, chopped
   ½ cup chopped pecans
      About ¼ cup plain low-fat yogurt

Bring water to a boil in medium saucepan. Stir in rice, margarine and, if desired, salt. Cover tightly and cook over low heat until all water is absorbed, about 50 minutes. Transfer to large bowl; cool to room temperature. Cover and chill. Combine honey and lemon juice. Add to rice; mix well. Stir in fruits and pecans. Add yogurt, as needed, to bind ingredients together. Cover and chill until ready to serve.   *Makes 10 servings*

Per Serving: 195 calories, 3 g protein, 5 g fat, 34 g carbohydrate, 230 mg sodium when prepared with salt

CREAMY RICE PUDDING

⅓ cup UNCLE BEN'S® CONVERTED® Brand Rice
1½ cups water
¼ cup sugar
1 teaspoon cornstarch
¼ teaspoon salt
1⅓ cups skim milk
2 teaspoons margarine
1 teaspoon vanilla
2 egg yolks, beaten
Ground cinnamon (optional)

Combine rice and water in medium saucepan. Bring to a boil. Reduce heat. Cover tightly and simmer 25 minutes, or until rice is very tender and most of water is absorbed. Combine sugar, cornstarch and salt. Add to rice with milk. Bring to a boil. Boil 1 minute, stirring constantly. Remove from heat. Stir in margarine and vanilla. Slowly stir about 1 cup of hot rice mixture into beaten egg yolks; blend with remaining mixture in saucepan. Cook over medium heat, stirring frequently, just until pudding starts to bubble. Serve warm or chilled, plain or sprinkled with cinnamon.

Makes 5 servings

Per Serving: 150 calories, 4 g protein, 4 g fat, 24 g carbohydrate, 163 mg sodium

ORANGE RICE DELIGHTS

   3 cups cooked rice*
   3 cups skim milk
   1 teaspoon grated orange peel
   ⅛ teaspoon salt (optional)
   1 package (0.3 ounces) artificially sweetened orange flavor gelatin
   1 teaspoon vanilla
   2 cups frozen non-dairy whipped topping, thawed
   2 oranges, peeled, sectioned, and coarsely chopped

Combine rice, milk, orange peel and, if desired, salt in medium saucepan. Bring to a boil. Reduce heat. Simmer 25 minutes or until thickened, stirring often. Add gelatin and vanilla; cool. Fold in whipped topping and oranges. Spoon into 12 individual ½-cup molds or one 6-cup mold. Chill until firm. Unmold onto serving plates. Garnish with additional whipped topping, if desired.
Makes 12 servings

*Prepared without butter or salt.

Per Serving: 115 calories, 4 g protein, 3 g fat, 18 g carbohydrate, 52 mg sodium when prepared without salt and served without additional whipped topping

BERRY GOOD YOGURT RICE PARFAITS

   1 cup UNCLE BEN'S® CONVERTED® Brand Rice
   2 cartons (8 ounces each) strawberry low-fat yogurt*
   2 cups sliced fresh strawberries
   Whole strawberries (optional)

Prepare rice according to package directions omitting butter and salt. Transfer to large bowl; cool to room temperature. Stir in yogurt. Cover and chill. Just before serving, layer rice mixture and strawberries in 8 parfait glasses or dessert dishes. Top with whole berries, if desired.

Makes 8 servings

*Blueberry or raspberry yogurt and fresh blueberries or raspberries may be substituted.

Per Serving: 155 calories, 4 g protein, 1 g fat, 32 g carbohydrate, 33 mg sodium when served without whole strawberries

PEACHY RICE DESSERT

2½ cups water
  1 cup UNCLE BEN'S® CONVERTED® Brand Rice
  1 package (3½ ounces) vanilla instant pudding and pie filling mix
2¼ cups skim milk
  1 carton (8 ounces) vanilla low-fat yogurt
  ½ teaspoon almond extract
  3 fresh peaches, peeled and thinly sliced*
  1 tablespoon toasted sliced almonds

Bring water to a boil in medium saucepan. Stir in rice. Cover tightly and simmer 20 minutes. Remove from heat. Let stand covered until all water is absorbed, about 5 minutes. Prepare pudding according to package directions, using 2¼ cups milk. Stir in rice, yogurt and almond extract. Layer rice mixture and peaches in 8 dessert glasses beginning and ending with rice mixture. Cover and chill. Garnish with almonds.

Makes 8 servings

*1 package (about 12 ounces) frozen unsweetened sliced peaches, thawed and drained, or 1 can (15 or 16 ounces) sliced peaches, packed in juice, drained, may be substituted.

Per Serving: 200 calories, 6 g protein, 1 g fat, 41 g carbohydrate, 212 mg sodium

INDEX

A
Aloha Rice Medley, 86
Apricot Brown Rice, 82
Arabian Rice Salad, 112
Arroz con Pollo Salad, 104

B
Barbecue Bonus Salad, 105
Beef and Rice Provencal, 61
Beef & Snow Peas Chinese-Style, 37
Berry Good Yogurt Rice Parfaits, 122
Broccoli Rice with Toasted Walnuts, 82
Brown Rice and Sprouts Oriental, 70
Brown Rice Chef's Salad Bowl, 97
Brown Rice Guadalajara, 79
Brown Rice Medley, 75
Brown Rice O'Brien, 90
Brown Rice Royal, 81

C
Calico Vegetable Rice Salad, 102
California Almond Pilaf, 87
Cantonese Chicken and Rice, 34
Caribbean Island Rice, 77
Casseroles: Charleston Rice, 74; Eggs Ranchero Brown Rice Casserole, 62; Mexican Turkey Bake, 41; Tri-Colored Salmon Bake, 59; Vegetarian Rice Bake (Rice Diet), 26
Charleston Rice, 74
Chicken: Arroz con Pollo Salad, 104; Cantonese Chicken and Rice, 34; Chicken and Rice Monterey, 40; Chicken Marengo, 46; Chicken Rice Salad Olé (Rice Diet), 22; Chicken Salad with Tarragon Vinaigrette, 116; Chicken with Pimiento Sauce over Green Rice, 31; Chinatown Chicken and Zucchini, 53; Curried Chicken Salad, 92; Curried Orange Chicken (Rice Diet), 18; Mexican Chicken with Jalapeño Rice, 51; Oriental Chicken Salad, 95; Pacific Paella, 32; Picante Chicken 'n Rice, 55; Polynesian Chicken and Rice, 57; Quick Chicken-Shrimp Gumbo, 48; Rosemary Chicken Kabobs, 42; Spicy Oriental Rice Salad, 107; Tarragon Chicken with California Rice, 45
Chili-Cheese Rice Quiche, 47
Chinatown Chicken and Zucchini, 53
Cioppino Rice Skillet, 40
Citrus Rice Cheesecake, 118
Citrusy Brown Rice Shrimp Salad, 100
Classic Pilaf, 74
Country Breakfast Cereal, 83
Country-Style Summer Vegetable Rice, 72
Creamy Rice Pudding, 121
Creole Fish 'n Rice Skillet, 63

Curried Chicken Salad, 92
Curried Orange Chicken (Rice Diet), 18
Curried Orange 'n Pear Rice, 72
Curried Summer Fruit 'n Brown Rice Salad, 106

D
Desserts: Berry Good Yogurt Rice Parfaits, 122; Creamy Rice Pudding, 121; Citrus Rice Cheesecake, 118; Fruit Treat, 120; Maple Walnut Rice Custard, 119; Mexican Chocolate Rice Cream (Rice Diet), 29; Orange Rice Delights, 122; Peachy Rice Dessert, 123; Pineapple Rice Bake, 120; Rice 'n Strawberry Pudding, 118
Dilly Cucumber Rice Salad, 112

E
Eggs: Chili-Cheese Rice Quiche, 47; Eggs Ranchero Brown Rice Casserole, 62; Fisherman's Frittata (Rice Diet), 28

F
Fiesta Thyme Rice, 75
Fish: Cioppino Rice Skillet, 40; Creole Fish 'n Rice Skillet, 63; Fish and Rice Marinara, 33; Fisherman's Frittata (Rice Diet), 28; Fish Kabobs & Zucchini Brown Rice, 56; Italian-Style Fish and Brown Rice Bake, 43; Lemon Fish and Rice Amandine, 34; Manhattan Style Fish Chowder (Rice Diet), 20; Monterey Fish and Brown Rice, 49; Nicoise Rice Salad, 94; Oriental Tuna Rice Salad (Rice Diet), 17; Sole Roll-Ups, 64; Sweet & Sour Tuna Salad, 100; Tri-Colored Salmon Bake, 59; Tuna and Brown Rice Salad, 108; Tuna Creole Skillet, 60
Fisherman's Frittata (Rice Diet), 28
Fruit-of-the-Season Rice Salad, 115
Fruits: Aloha Rice Medley, 86; Apricot Brown Rice, 82; Berry Good Yogurt Rice Parfaits, 122; Caribbean Island Rice, 77; Curried Orange 'n Pear Rice, 72; Curried Summer Fruit 'n Brown Rice Salad, 106; Fruit-of-the-Season Rice Salad, 115; Fruit Treat, 120; Hawaiian Turkey Salad, 113; Orange Rice Delights, 122; Peachy Rice Dessert, 123; Pineapple Rice Bake, 120; Rice 'n Strawberry Pudding, 118; Summer's Special Brown Rice Fruit Salad, 108; Sunshine Rice Salad, 96; Three Fruit Rice Salad (Rice Diet), 24; Three Melon Rice Salad, 111; Waldorf-Style Rice, 78

G
Garden Vegetable Pilaf, 89
Garden Vegetable Rice Salad, 96
Garden Vegetable Saute with Brown Rice, 70
Gazpacho-Style Rice, 68
Gingered Pork and Pea Pods (Rice Diet), 23
Gingered Shrimp and Spring Rice, 58
Grecian Spinach Rice, 88
Green Peppers Stuffed with Mediterranean Rice, 78
Green Rice, 84
Gulf Coast Salad, 93
Gypsy Fried Rice, 39

Index 125

H
Harvest Rice, 67
Hawaiian Turkey Salad, 113
Herbed Vegetable Rice, 86

I
Italian Rice Salad, 92
Italian-Style Fish and Brown Rice Bake, 43

J
Jambalaya Rice Salad, 109

L
Lemon Fish and Rice Amandine, 34
Lemon Veal Chops with Herbed Rice (Rice Diet), 19
Lemony Zucchini Brown Rice, 66

M
Manhattan Style Fish Chowder (Rice Diet), 20
Maple Walnut Rice Custard, 119
Marinated Shrimp Kabobs with Confetti Rice, 44
Meal-In-One Salad, 114
Meats: Beef and Rice Provencal, 61; Beef & Snow Peas Chinese-Style, 37; Gingered Pork and Pea Pods (Rice Diet), 23; Gypsy Fried Rice, 39; Jambalaya Rice Salad, 109; Lemon Veal Chops with Herbed Rice (Rice Diet), 19; Oriental Vegetable and Lamb Skillet, 60; Pacific Paella, 32; Rice Salad Italia, 114; San Francisco Pork Fried Rice, 54
Mexican Chicken with Jalapeño Rice, 51
Mexican Chocolate Rice Cream (Rice Diet), 29
Mexican Turkey Bake, 41
Middle Eastern Pilaf, 68
Mixed Vegetable Curry and Spicy Rice, 38
Monterey Fish and Brown Rice, 49
Monterey Risotto, 71

N
Nicoise Rice Salad, 94

O
Orange Rice Delights, 122
Oriental Chicken Salad, 95
Oriental Rice Pilaf, 73
Oriental Tuna Rice Salad (Rice Diet), 17
Oriental Vegetable and Lamb Skillet, 60

P
Pacific Paella, 32
Parmesan Eggplant Skillet, 76
Peachy Rice Dessert, 123
Peppery Brown Rice & Tomato Salad, 99
Picante Chicken 'n Rice, 55
Pilaf: California Almond Pilaf, 87; Classic Pilaf, 74; Garden Vegetable Pilaf, 89; Middle Eastern Pilaf, 68; Oriental Rice Pilaf, 73
Pineapple Rice Bake, 120
Polynesian Chicken and Rice, 57

Q
Quick Chicken-Shrimp Gumbo, 48
Quick 'n Easy Ratatouille Rice (Rice Diet), 27

R
Rice Fontina Salad, 101
Rice 'n Strawberry Pudding, 118
Rice Salad Italia, 114
Rice Salad Milano, 104
Risotto: Monterey Risotto, 71; Risotto alla Milanese, 81; Risotto alla Napolitana, 76; Risotto with Garden Vegetables, 84; White Risotto with Mushrooms, 66

Rosemary Chicken Kabobs, 42

S
Salads, accompaniment: Arabian Rice Salad, 112; Barbecue Bonus Salad, 105; Calico Vegetable Rice Salad, 102; Curried Summer Fruit 'n Brown Rice Salad, 106; Dilly Cucumber Rice Salad, 112; Fruit-of-the-Season Rice Salad, 115; Garden Vegetable Rice Salad, 96; Italian Rice Salad, 92; Peppery Brown Rice & Tomato Salad, 99; Rice Fontina Salad, 101; Rice Salad Milano, 104; Spinach Salad with Oriental Vinaigrette, 103; Summer's Special Brown Rice Fruit Salad, 108; Sunshine Rice Salad, 96; Three Fruit Rice Salad (Rice Diet), 24; Three Melon Rice Salad, 111; Vegetable Medley Salad with Sherry Dressing, 98
Salads, main dish: Arroz con Pollo Salad, 104; Brown Rice Chef's Salad Bowl, 97; Chicken Rice Salad Olé (Rice Diet), 22; Chicken Salad with Tarragon Vinaigrette, 116; Citrusy Brown Rice Shrimp Salad, 100; Curried Chicken Salad, 92; Gulf Coast Salad, 93; Hawaiian Turkey Salad, 113; Jambalaya Rice Salad, 109; Meal-In-One Salad, 114; Nicoise Rice Salad, 94; Oriental Chicken Salad, 95; Oriental Tuna Rice Salad (Rice Diet), 17; Rice Salad Italia, 114; Seafood Salad with Orange Vinaigrette, 110; Spicy Oriental Rice Salad, 107; Sweet & Sour Tuna Salad, 100; Tuna and Brown Rice Salad, 108
San Francisco Pork Fried Rice, 54
Scallop Saute with Curried Rice, 52
Scallop Stir Fry, 36
Seafood Salad with Orange Vinaigrette, 110
Sesame Zucchini Rice, 88
Shellfish: Cioppino Rice Skillet, 40; Citrusy Brown Rice Shrimp Salad, 100; Gingered Shrimp and Spring Rice, 58; Gulf Coast Salad, 93; Jambalaya Rice Salad, 109; Marinated Shrimp Kabobs with Confetti Rice, 44; Pacific Paella, 32; Quick Chicken-Shrimp Gumbo, 48; Scallop Saute with Curried Rice, 52; Scallop Stir Fry, 36; Seafood Salad with Orange Vinaigrette, 110; Shrimp and Rice Veracruz, 54; Shrimp Fried Rice, 50; South of the Border Shrimpy Rice (Rice Diet), 25
Shrimp and Rice Veracruz, 54
Shrimp Fried Rice, 50
Slim Spanish Rice (Rice Diet), 21
Sole Roll-Ups, 64
Soups: Manhattan Style Fish Chowder (Rice Diet), 20; Quick Chicken-Shrimp Gumbo, 48; Turkey Oriental Soup, 50
South of the Border Shrimpy Rice (Rice Diet), 25
Southwestern Rice, 85
Spicy Oriental Rice Salad, 107
Spinach Salad with Oriental Vinaigrette, 103
Spring Garden Brown Rice Supper, 35
Summer's Special Brown Rice Fruit Salad, 108

Sunshine Rice Salad, 96
Sweet & Sour Tuna Salad, 100

T
Tarragon Chicken with California Rice, 45
Three Fruit Rice Salad (Rice Diet), 24
Three Melon Rice Salad, 111
Tomato Rice Ring Italian-Style, 80
Tri-Colored Salmon Bake, 59
Tuna and Brown Rice Salad, 108
Tuna Creole Skillet, 60
Turkey: Brown Rice Chef's Salad Bowl, 97; Chicken Salad with Tarragon Vinaigrette, 116; Hawaiian Turkey Salad, 113; Mexican Turkey Bake, 41; Spicy Oriental Rice Salad, 107; Turkey Oriental Soup, 50

V
Vegetable Brown Rice Curry, 69
Vegetable Medley Salad with Sherry Dressing, 98
Vegetables: Broccoli Rice with Toasted Walnuts, 82; Brown Rice and Sprouts Oriental, 70; Brown Rice Guadalajara, 79; Brown Rice Medley, 75; Country-Style Summer Vegetable Rice, 72; Fiesta Thyme Rice, 75; Garden Vegetable Saute with Brown Rice, 70; Gazpacho-Style Rice, 68; Grecian Spinach Rice, 88; Green Peppers Stuffed with Mediterranean Rice, 78; Green Rice, 84; Harvest Rice, 67; Herbed Vegetable Rice, 86; Lemony Zucchini Brown Rice, 66; Mixed Vegetable Curry and Spicy Rice, 38; Parmesan Eggplant Skillet, 76; Quick 'n Easy Ratatouille Rice (Rice Diet), 27; Sesame Zucchini Rice, 88; Slim Spanish Rice (Rice Diet), 21; Spring Garden Brown Rice Supper, 35; Tomato Rice Ring Italian-Style, 80; Vegetable Brown Rice Curry, 69; Vegetarian Rice Bake (Rice Diet), 26

W
Waldorf-Style Rice, 78
West Coast Raisin Rice, 90
Western Beans and Rice, 46
White Risotto with Mushrooms, 66